Pregnancy & Childbirth
Everything You Need To Know From Conception To Labor And Delivery

Table of Contents

About the Book 3

About the Author 4

Introduction 6

Chapter 1 – Discovering You're Pregnant 8

    Diagnosing Pregnancy 8

    Signs & Symptoms of Pregnancy 10

    Pregnancy Timeline 11

    Calculating Your Due Date 12

Chapter 2 – Knowing What To Do Next 14

    Choosing Your Physician 14

    Patient-Practitioner Relationship 16

Chapter 3 – Medications, Screenings, Tests & Procedures During Pregnancy 18

    Medications 18

    Screening Tests 18

Chapter 4 – Food & Pregnancy – What's Right & Wrong 23

    Prenatal Vitamins 23

    Benefits Of Pregnancy Diet 24

    Rules Of Healthy Pregnancy Eating 25

    What Foods To Eat & How Much 27

Chapter 5 – The First Trimester 32

    The First Prenatal Visit 32

    Month 1 32

    Month 2 33

    Month 3 34

Chapter 6 – The Second Trimester 35

    Month 4 35

    Month 5 36

    Month 6 38

Chapter 7 – The Third Trimester 40

    Month 7 40

    Month 8 42

Month 9 43

Chapter 8 – Childbirth – What You Need To Know 46

    Stage One – Labor 46

        Phase One – Early Labor 47

        Phase Two – Active Labor 48

        Phase Three – Transitional Labor 49

    Stage Two – Delivery of the Baby 50

    Stage Three – Delivery of the Placenta 52

Chapter 9 – What To Avoid When Pregnant 54

    Alcohol Consumption 54

    Tobacco Use 55

    Drug Use – From Marijuana To Cocaine & Everything In Between 57

    Caffeine Use 57

    Sugar Substitutes 58

    Hot Tubs, Saunas & Electric Blankets 58

Chapter 10 – Q&A 60

    When Is A C-Section Necessary? 60

    What Does Rh Negative/Positive Mean? 61

    Is Making Love While Pregnant Safe? 62

    What Medications Are Used For Pain Relief During Labor? 63

    What Causes Premature Labor & Can You Prevent It? 65

    Is Exercising While Pregnant Important? 66

    What Is The Effect Of Cell Phone Use During Pregnancy? 67

    What Is Preeclampsia? 68

    What Should You Know About Miscarriage? 69

    Are Household Cleaning Products Safe To Use During Pregnancy? 70

    What Is Gestational Diabetes? 72

    What Are The Benefits Of Breastfeeding? 73

    Weight Gain During Pregnancy – What You Need To Know 75

    How Do You Know If You're Having Twins? 77

About the Book

This book is a guide to pregnancy from conception to birth and everything in between. You will learn about methods for diagnosing pregnancy, tests used to determine how your baby is developing and the importance of communicating with your practitioner. You will also discover the importance of the pregnancy diet, prenatal vitamins and what things should be avoided during pregnancy, from tobacco and alcohol use to the use of illegal substances and caffeine, all of which pose negative risk factors for the development of your baby.

You will also be provided with an outline of the next nine months of your life, including what you may be feeling emotionally and mentally, reassuring you that crying over spilled milk during pregnancy is often acceptable. Further, there is information on what you may be experiencing physically, from being exhausted and having to constantly pee to feeling nauseous and constipated all in the same day, again reassuring you that this is perfectly normal.

The goal of this book is to provide you with the information you need to conduct a safe and healthy pregnant environment for your baby to grow and develop in. It is not meant, however, to scare you out of your mind with the different complications that can occur during pregnancy. If at any time you are reading this and you begin feeling overwhelmed by the information or are unsure about anything, ask your practitioner. After all, you chose this individual because of their expertise and experience in the field of pregnancy.

With that said, sit back, put your feet up and enjoy learning about the life you should live for the next nine months while there is a child growing inside you, completely dependent on you taking care of them. Relaxation, rest, adequate nutrition and fluid intake are essential. So, grab a glass of water, read a few pages, take a nap, read a few more and become the best pregnant mom you can be! Oh, and don't forget to go pee, because it's likely you need to after reading this introduction, even though you just went five minutes ago!

About the Author

As the mother of two beautiful and amazing young children – an almost 6-year old son and a 4-year old daughter – and an aunt to many gorgeous girls, with another niece – or perhaps a nephew – on the way, I know all about pregnancy.

You see, more than nine years ago, I was in the room with my sister when the first of our younger generation was born. Birth is an amazing experience, albeit somewhat scary. My niece had the umbilical cord wrapped around her neck and was having troubles. Only seconds before an emergency C-section was conducted, did my sister's obstetrician save the day, by flipping the umbilical cord from around her neck.

My own experience was slightly more scary. When I had my son almost six years ago, everything was going great – the pregnancy was healthy, I was healthy, our baby boy was healthy. My delivery was scheduled for May 3 – I was being induced. Everything seemed to be going well and about an hour into the induction, I needed something for the pain – at this time in my life I was kind of wimpy – so they did an epidural and moved me to the delivery room.

After hours of pain and agony, even with the epidural, my doctor came in again to check on me. After my obstetrician tried to stretch my cervix and use a vacuum to suck my son out, as my cervix was not dilating, she decided to wait a little longer to see if that would help.

Unfortunately, not much later, the nurses were having trouble finding our baby's heartbeat and my husband and I were scared – why is it hurting? where is the heartbeat? is everything going to be okay? – these were the questions running through our minds. My obstetrician came back in and she declared an emergency C-section was necessary – no other options.

Having only been married a short time, and this being our first baby, my husband was scared and he wasn't allowed to come in with me. My doctor and nurses moved me quickly – I don't even remember getting to say I love you my husband – and he had to sign papers, choosing between my life and the baby's. It was awful. The last thing I remembered before being put under anesthetics was hearing my obstetrician tell the girls to scrub in – my baby had no heartbeat, or at least one they could find.

After a period of time – I really have no clue how long, due to the medications – everything was fine – my baby boy was healthy and so was I. What had apparently happened, was when my obstetrician broke my water, his little bum molded to my uterus and the pain I kept feeling was him trying to make his way out the birth canal with my uterus! But everything was perfect in the world again – we were together – our family of three, thanks to the amazing quick decision-making of my obstetrician and her team!

A year later, we were blessed with another baby – a girl, but this time we scheduled a C-section, so that I could be awake and my husband could hold my hand. During this delivery, we also opted to have a tubal ligation performed, as our family as now complete – two boys & two girls.

Pregnancy and childbirth is a beautiful thing. Having the knowledge you need to carry a healthy baby to full term and keep yourself healthy in the process, is what this book is meant to provide. I have background information on a variety of topics, from either my own experience or from being a part of someone's journey who is close to me. This includes vaginal births, cesarean sections, infections after surgery, tubal ligations, miscarriages, and more. Everything has been included in this book for your benefit.

I think knowing about what is important in pregnancy and what you can expect as you progress through your pregnancy is how healthy babies are made. While not everything is in our hands – our faith is a lot of it – we need to do our part as mother's to protect our children from the moment we know they are on the way!

You are probably only looking at this book because either you or someone close to you is pregnant. So, I want to take the time to raise my glass with you – glass of milk that is – and say congratulations and here's to a happy, healthy, safe pregnancy and the birth of your baby!

Introduction

Pregnancy is a very vast medical condition, featuring a wide variety of risks, complications, rules and regulations, and in the end a reward. However, because pregnancy has so many subtopics associated with it, it can be quite overwhelming for an individual who is pregnant, especially for the first time. However, becoming educated about pregnancy is the first step to having a healthy pregnancy.

A lot has changed since your grandmother and even your mother were both pregnant. This book is designed to give you the basic information you need during pregnancy, what you should be concerned about and how to communicate with your practitioner. There is no one right answer for every pregnancy and every expecting individual. This book serves as a guideline to what is normally seen during pregnancy.

Chapter one focuses on methods for diagnosing pregnancy and the signs and symptoms of pregnancy that might lead you to suspect you might be pregnant. In this chapter, you will also learn about the pregnancy timeline and how a due date is calculated, although the only person who really knows when your baby will be born is your baby.

In chapter two, you will learn about choosing your practitioner, as there are many types available. You will also discover how important communication with your practitioner is in having a safe and healthy pregnancy.

Chapter three brings to light some of the different screenings, tests and procedures conducted during pregnancy, as well as the importance of discussing medications with your practitioner. Although this section does not encompass all possible methods and tests used to detect certain things during pregnancy, it does provide you with a background of what you could possibly expect to need – test-wise – during pregnancy.

The focus of chapter four is food. While there are many old wives' tales centered around ice cream and pickle sundaes, this is not necessarily what you should be eating while you are pregnant. There are a variety of foods that provide the nutrition needed to keep you and your baby safe and provide adequate nutrition for the development of your baby. It is important that you understand what these foods provide and that you also incorporate them into your diet. There is also a section on prenatal vitamins, as they are an important part of the pregnancy diet.

Chapters five, six and seven are a guide to pregnancy month by month. Chapter five takes into account what you will experience physically, emotionally and mentally during the first trimester. Chapter six focuses on the months of the second trimester, getting you to the halfway point of your pregnancy, and chapter seven discusses the third trimester, which leads you to labor and delivery. You will also learn information about how your baby should be developing at the end of each month and what is to come for your baby in the following months.

Childbirth is what you will learn about in chapter eight. There is a lot about childbirth that can be interesting to learn about and is important to know. This chapter, however, is not meant to scare you or make you nervous about having a baby. There are a lot of things involved in delivery, from the use of medications for anesthesia – epidurals and spinal taps – to medications used for induction of labor. The simplest way to prepare for childbirth is to discuss your wants, needs and concerns about the event with your practitioner months in advance. This will help relieve your stress about delivery day and answer any questions you have, making sure you and your practitioner are on the same page.

As with any medical condition, and yes pregnancy is a medical condition, there are many things you should avoid coming in contact with or using during pregnancy. Chapter nine focuses on many of these subjects, from tobacco and alcohol use to caffeine and electric blanket use. It is important that you do nothing you are wary of without first discussing it with your physician.

Because pregnancy is such a vast medical condition, not every question can be answered in a book, unless that book has hundreds or thousands of pages and was written by an OB-GYN himself/herself. However, there are a few additional questions that many women are concerned about during pregnancy, wherein the answers can be found in chapter ten.

It is important, however, to remember that any time you are feeling unsure about something, whether it's eating a particular food or having a procedure conducted that was recommended by your practitioner, it is important that you discuss your apprehension and feelings with your practitioner. The key to a healthy pregnancy is this book, of course, excellent communication between you and your physician, following the pregnancy diet and reliving yourself from stress and focusing on you and your baby for the next nine months, or 40 weeks, however you look at it!

Chapter 1 – Discovering You're Pregnant

You missed your period last month, and thought maybe it was stress, or just you being stir occasionally busy. However, this month things have calmed down, but you're a day late, then a week late and you start thinking – am I pregnant? There are a lot of things to consider when you think you're pregnant, from how can you be sure you are pregnant to what you need to do next.

Diagnosing Pregnancy

First, you need to figure out whether or not you really are pregnant. There are a variety of different tests that can be conducted to determine if you are pregnant and sometimes, how far along you are. These include the home pregnancy test, an in-office urine test, a blood test and a medical exam.

Home Pregnancy Test

The most common test for pregnancy is the home urine test. Many women select this option prior to having another test done by their doctor. Home pregnancy tests can be purchased at your local pharmacy or supermarket. Here's what you need to know about home pregnancy tests.

A home pregnancy test is a urine test, similar to those conducted by physicians, wherein the test determines whether or not you are pregnant by measuring the level of the hCG (human chorionic gonadotropin) hormone, also known as the pregnancy hormone, levels in your urine. Typically, home pregnancy tests are completed in a few minutes and can be conducted within 14 days of conception using urine at any time of the day.

However, it is recommended that you test your urine using a home pregnancy test first thing in the morning and wait until you are about one week late with your period. When it comes to accuracy, a home pregnancy test can be as accurate as one conducted by your doctor, as long as it was performed correctly.

Home pregnancy tests offer two different advantages – privacy and immediate results. Further, because you typically take a home pregnancy test sooner than you would make an appointment with your physician, you can begin getting the proper care you need faster.

On the other hand, home pregnancy tests can be expensive and are not covered by medical insurance. Also, depending on how you feel about the test, you may not be confident in the results and want to re-test, spending even more money.

Probably even more important when it comes to the drawbacks of home pregnancy tests is that they can often produce false negatives. This means that the test can read negative but you are actually pregnant, which could postpone the time it takes you to get to a physician and obtain proper prenatal care.

When using an at-home pregnancy test, it is important that you understand that it is not designed to take the place of a test conducted by your physician. You should always follow up with your physician after taking an at-home pregnancy test, whether the test is positive or negative. This means that if the result is positive, you should check with your physician about confirming the pregnancy and begin prenatal care, starting with a checkup. In the event that it reads negative, you should still consult with your physician, to make sure that it is not a false negative, stir occasionally that you still get the prenatal care you need.

Further, while you are waiting to meet with your physician to confirm whether or not you are pregnant, it is a good idea to avoid things that can harm an unborn child. This includes cigarettes and alcohol, to name a few.

Physician-Conducted Urine Pregnancy Test

The second type of test used to determine whether or not you are pregnant is similar to the first, except the urine test is conducted in your physician's office. It also detects the levels of hCG in your urine, but does so with near 100% accuracy, and can be conducted anywhere between 7 and 14 days following conception.

Different from the home pregnancy test, the physician-conducted urine pregnancy test is theoretically more accurate, as the person performing the test is a professional. A pregnancy urine test conducted by a physician's office does not require that your urine be from the first pee of the morning. You can urinate at any time of the day for this test to be conducted.

While this type of urine pregnancy test does cost more than an at-home test, it is often covered by your health insurance. Further, the physician-conducted urine test is less expensive than a blood test, but does not provide as much vital information about your pregnancy.

Blood Pregnancy Test

The blood pregnancy test can determine whether or not you are pregnant with nearly 100% accuracy as early as one week after conception. The blood test is conducted in the same manner that any other type of blood test and is taken from the veins in the arm.

Unlike urine pregnancy tests, the blood pregnancy test can give your physician more information about your pregnancy, such as the exact date of conception, which enables the physician to determine a more exact due date. This is done by calculating the exact hCG levels in the blood, which change as your pregnancy progresses. In many cases, a physician will order both the urine pregnancy test and the blood pregnancy test. This enables them to be sure they are making the correct diagnosis of pregnancy.

Medical Exam

Whether you choose an at-home pregnancy test, a physician-conducted urine pregnancy test or a blood pregnancy test, the validity of the diagnosis can become more concrete through a medical exam. There are physical signs of pregnancy, such as a softened uterus and a change in the texture of the cervix, that are apparent to many physicians during a physical medical exam. This can take place and be accurate anywhere from 4-6 weeks of conception.

When your physician conducts the medical exam, he/she is looking for a few particular signs and symptoms of pregnancy. This includes changes in the color of vaginal tissue, softening of the cervix and/or uterus, an enlarged uterus and abdomen, and a palpable uterine artery pulsation. These signs are what lead to a diagnosis of pregnancy as the result of a medical exam.

As is the case with pregnancy tests, the physician's diagnosis of pregnant is more likely to be correct that a diagnosis of not pregnant. With that said, you should know that statistically, false negatives are very rare when a full medical exam is conducted.

Signs & Symptoms of Pregnancy

Aside from missing your period, there are several other signs and symptoms of pregnancy that can occur at different times during the pregnancy. It is important to understand that these are just some signs and symptoms commonly experienced during pregnancy.

This does not mean, however that if you have none of these symptoms that it is safe to assume that you are not pregnant. Further, it also does not mean that if you have all of these signs and symptoms that it is safe to assume you are pregnant.

Every pregnancy is different and every person is different. Therefore, it is obvious that every sign and symptom for each individual will be different. With that said, it is important that you pay attention to these common signs and symptoms and discuss any symptoms that you experience with your physician.

Possible Signs & Symptoms of Pregnancy

For many, about 50% of women to be exact, morning sickness is a common symptom during the first 2-8 weeks after conception. You may experience nausea, with or without vomiting. Further, although the name has been given to this symptom of morning sickness, this can actually occur at any time during the day.

As you progress through your pregnancy you will likely experience frequent urination. This can happen as early as two weeks after conception and typically continues or becomes worse as you reach childbirth.

Other symptoms you may experience include tingling, swollen, tender breasts, as early as a few days after conception. You may also notice, sometime during the first trimester of pregnancy, that the area around your nipples has become darker, and you will likely notice elevation of tiny glands around the nipples.

The first trimester has some other symptoms that may appear as well. For instance, you may begin noticing blue and pink lines underneath your skin near your breasts, which can later progress to your abdomen. Also, during the first trimester, you may experience food cravings, which could be your body telling you that you are lacking certain vitamins and minerals.

Lastly, sometime around the fourth or fifth month of pregnancy, you may begin to notice a line developing from your bellybutton to your pubis. This line is known as linea nigra, and is often very dark.

Probable Signs & Symptoms of Pregnancy

Aside from what your physician looks for during a medical exam to conclude a diagnosis, there is one more sign that is almost always related to pregnancy – fluttering in your abdomen. This is a result of the fetus moving around in your uterus. If you are feeling these types of sensations and have any of the other signs and symptoms of pregnancy, you should discuss this with your physician if you have not.

Positive Signs & Symptoms of Pregnancy

There are some things that everyone will experience during pregnancy and are 100% related to and can only be caused by pregnancy. This is a visualization of the embryo developing in the uterus, which is done by an ultrasound conducted by your physician as early as 4-6 weeks following conception.

The other 100% positive sign of pregnancy is hearing the heartbeat of the fetus. The heart is typically able to be heard anywhere from 10-20 weeks of pregnancy.

There are no other explanations for these two signs and symptoms of pregnancy, and therefore, mean that you are indeed pregnant!

Pregnancy Timeline

Typically, it is said that you are pregnant for nine months, but a healthcare professional actually classifies pregnancy time based on weeks, not months. This is because you are typically pregnant for 40 weeks, which could technically be considered 10 months. This is where it also gets confusing.

The 40 weeks take into account the first day of your last period. However, ovulation and conception don't actually occur for another three weeks, meaning you actually become pregnant in the third week of your pregnancy.

Although this can be very confusing, as you are not actually pregnant when the pregnancy clock starts, as you progress through your pregnancy, things may begin making a little more sense. You will reach certain milestones based on the number of weeks you are pregnant. For instance, the baby's heartbeat can be heard around 10 weeks and the top of the uterus will be near your bellybutton around 20 weeks.

Further, there are three different sections, called trimesters, of pregnancy. The first trimester takes into account activity during the first 1-13 weeks, the second trimester accounts for weeks 14-27 and the third trimester makes up for weeks 28-40. Each trimester brings about different experiences during pregnancy, which will be discussed in later chapters.

Calculating Your Due Date

If you or a healthcare professional have determined that you are pregnant, one of the first things women think about is their due date, so they can begin planning for the arrival of the baby. There are a few different ways a healthcare professional can calculate the due date, meaning when the baby will be born.

Unfortunately, it is important that you realize that the due date is only an estimate and babies come when babies want to come. This is probably why the due date is also known as the EDD – estimated date of delivery.

With that said, if this is the first time you are pregnant, your due date is typically set somewhere between week 40 and week 41 of your pregnancy. Your healthcare professional will calculate the due date using a simple calculation – subtract three months from the date of your last menstrual period and then add seven days. That will provide you with the due date for your baby.

To help you understand this a little more, if the first date of your last menstrual period began on April 10, you would count backwards three months, landing on January 10. Then, you need to add seven days, bringing your due date to January 17.

Unfortunately, not every woman has regular periods and not every woman keeps track of their menstrual cycles – although they should. Therefore, this method of calculation is not always an option. However, because an EDD is an important part of your pregnancy, for both you and your healthcare physician, there are other methods that provide clues to this day.

First, is the size of your uterus, which will be determined during your internal physical exam conducted when you discover you are pregnant. The size of your uterus should match up with what you believe is the date of conception and how far along you are in your pregnancy.

As you progress through your pregnancy, other milestones typically occur at certain weeks of the pregnancy, helping to secure the pregnancy timeline to your due date. For instance, the baby's heartbeat is typically heard between week 10 and week 12 using a Doppler device, and can then be heard using a stethoscope around 18 to 20 weeks.

Further, you will begin to notice the baby moving about in your uterus at about 20 to 22 weeks, causing a feeling of butterflies in your stomach. Also, at around 20 weeks, the top of your uterus, known as the fundus, will be at your bellybutton. This is not something you will necessarily notice or realize, but your healthcare professional will.

If these instances occur in line with the due date you and your practitioner have calculated, it is safe to assume that your due date is pretty close to accurate. However, this does not mean that the baby will definitely, positively, 100% come on the due date. This is an estimated time of delivery, and many factors can change when a baby is born.

With that said, your physician can and may conduct an ultrasound around 12 weeks to further determine if the chosen due date is still correct. This is done by taking a look at the size of the fetus. Also, as you progress closer to the end of your pregnancy, other clues can lead your physician to agree to or alter the due date.

For instance, minor contractions, the fetus dropping into the pelvis, which is known as engagement, your cervix becoming thinner, which is known as effacement, and the dilation of your cervix. As these symptoms develop, you can be sure you are closer to delivery. However, as was said before and often needs to be said again, no one knows with 100% guarantee when your delivery date will be, except your baby.

Chapter 2 – Knowing What To Do Next

Now that you have discovered that you are and have been diagnosed with being pregnant, you may be wondering, what's next. There are a lot of things you need to do to prepare to have a child. However, the most important thing you need to do is make an appointment to see a healthcare professional who specializes in pregnancy.

Choosing Your Physician

Prenatal care is the most valuable things you can provide your baby with at this point in his/her life. As soon as you discover that you are pregnant, call to make an appointment – do not delay. You may be wondering, however, just whom you should make an appointment with. If you already have a physician, such as an OB-GYN, you should give them a call. If not, it is important that you understand the differences between the types of people who can aide in your care during pregnancy and childbirth. This will help you make a decision about who to call.

There are three different types of professionals who can care for you during pregnancy and childbirth – an obstetrician, a family practitioner and/or a nurse-midwife. Each one will be explored in detail, so that you can determine who you will choose.

Obstetrician

An obstetrician, also called an OB-GYN, is a trained professional, who has the ability to answer all of your questions, no matter how strange they may seem. Further, an obstetrician is trained to handle your entire pregnancy, including the labor and delivery of your baby and any post-partum (after pregnancy) care you should need.

Further, an obstetrician can also provide other medical care for you when you are not pregnant, such as performing your annual pap smear exam, conducting breast exams and any other female health issues you may have.

In the case of a high-risk pregnancy, you should consider choosing an obstetrician, or even an obstetrician who specializes in high-risk pregnancies. This person is also likely to be certified in maternal and fetal medicine.

However, if your pregnancy seems to be progressing normally, you can choose any obstetrician to care for you. Although there are different types of professionals who can provide prenatal and delivery services, 80% of women still choose an obstetrician.

Make sure when you choose someone that they are a professional you trust, have heard good things about and someone you are comfortable talking with. One of the most important aspects of a healthy pregnancy is being able to talk with your physician about anything.

Family Practitioner

Next on the list of professionals who can provide prenatal and delivery services is the family practitioner. After receiving a medical degree (MD), these individuals go on to obtain training in obstetrics, pediatrics and primary care. Although not many women take this route, only about 12%, they are still qualified to care for you during pregnancy.

Further, you can choose to have this individual care for your child once he/she is born, serving as their pediatrician. Having a family practitioner for your pregnancy may be a good idea, especially if you want to keep one doctor for the whole family.

In the event that any type of problems arise during your pregnancy, it is likely that a family practitioner will refer you to an obstetrician. Many times, however, when this event occurs, your family practitioner will stay on to be a part of caring for you and your baby.

Certified Nurse-Midwife

Although not many women choose them, only about 9% of pregnant women, a certified nurse-midwife can serve as your healthcare professional during pregnancy and birth. A certified nurse-midwife focuses on you as a person, rather than as a patient. Typically, a nurse-midwife will spend a lot of time talking to you about more than just your pregnancy, such as how you're feeling mentally and physically, and to help you cope with any problems, or stresses you are having during pregnancy.

A certified nurse-midwife is a registered nurse who continued her education by taking graduate-level courses in midwifery and has been certified through the American College of Nurse-Midwives.

With that said, due to the type of training they receive, nurse-midwives are only capable of handling uncomplicated pregnancies and uncomplicated births. Some nurse-midwives can also provide care to your newborn and continuing gynecological care for you.

When it comes to the actual delivery of your baby, with a nurse-midwife, you have more options, as opposed to an obstetrician who performs deliveries in the hospital only. A nurse-midwife may work at the hospital, a birthing center and sometimes can perform delivery in the comfort of your own home.

If you are searching for an individual who really believes in having natural births, a certified nurse-midwife may be right for you. A natural birth is one without medications, such as epidurals and other pain medications, to relive the pains of giving birth. With that said, however, many nurse-midwives are eligible, depending on the state in which they practice, to prescribe pain medications.

When it comes to choosing between a nurse-midwife and an obstetrician, you should know that research has proven that a birth conducted by a nurse-midwife, providing it is a low-risk pregnancy and birth – is just as safe as one conducted by an obstetrician. Further, many certified nurse-midwives work directly with an obstetrician in the event that a complication arises during the pregnancy or the birth.

If you are interested in choosing a nurse-midwife, talk to one to see what their plans for your pregnancy are, where they delivery, what types of medications, if any, do they prescribe and whether or not they work with obstetricians as a backup plan.

Direct-Entry Midwives

The last type of healthcare professional that could assist in your care during pregnancy and childbirth is a direct-entry midwife. Although she is not a nurse, a direct-entry midwife has training to care for you during pregnancy and childbirth. Further, she will likely have a degree in other medical fields.

A direct-entry midwife that has been certified by the North American Registry of Midwives are often referred to as Certified Professional Midwives, where other direct-entry midwives are not certified. Some states do provide licenses for direct-entry midwives who are not certified and some types of private health insurance and Medicaid do provide reimbursement for these individuals. However, there are some states that do not legally permit direct entry midwives to practice.

A direct-entry midwife will be more likely to perform an at-home birth than any other medical professional. If this is something you are interested, you should contact the Midwives Alliance of North America for more details on the rules and regulations about midwives in your state.

Patient-Practitioner Relationship

No matter which type of practitioner you choose, it is a good idea to have an excellent relationship with that individual. This can be accomplished through excellent communication between you and your practitioner.

It is important that you ask questions about your pregnancy, no matter how silly they seem. However, it's not a good idea to call with every pain you feel, unless it is extreme or unable to be a cause of something you ate, or something along those lines. It is important that if you are unsure of anything that you do call your practitioner. Having good communication is the key to a successful pregnancy.

During your pregnancy, you will likely hear a lot of opinions of others about what you should and should not do and eat during pregnancy. Talking these opinions over with your physician, especially if it is the exact opposite of what he/she told you, is an excellent idea. They may be able to tell you why some people think one thing while they think another. This doesn't me you go storming in their office and confront them in a negative fashion. It simply means that if you are concerned about something, you discuss it with your practitioner.

In addition, it is important that you are completely, 100% honest with your practitioner. Do not give them an incomplete, incorrect or false family or personal history regarding anything. The only way they can provide you with proper care, and be able to keep an eye out for any possible complications is by knowing everything about you, your health and your habits. This includes the use of any illegal or recreational drugs, alcoholic beverages, medications and tobacco use that you are currently using or taking or have done so recently. What you and your physician discuss is confidential. They cannot and will not tell anyone what you discuss without your permission.

If you are unsure of anything your practitioner is telling you at any point during your pregnancy, be sure to ask for further explanations. A good practitioner will be willing to explain anything until you are able to comprehend the concept. This is especially true when it comes to different tests your practitioner may recommend, which will be discussed in detail in a later chapter.

You should also alert your practitioner to any oddities, such as uncommon symptoms that you experience during your pregnancy. This could be anything from an adverse reaction to a medication to bleeding, even if only slightly, during pregnancy. It is very important that your physician be aware of what's going on when you are not in the office.

You should be able to trust your practitioner and take his/her advice when it comes to different tests, medications, procedures and the delivery of your baby. Make sure you listen to what he/she is saying, ask questions and most of all, follow their advice. They are the professionals and know what you need. This is especially true when it comes to attending appointments, going on bed rest, if necessary, getting the right amount of exercise, the pregnancy diet, medications and so forth.

Chapter 3 – Medications, Screenings, Tests & Procedures During Pregnancy

Now that you have chosen the right practitioner for you and your baby, there are some things you need to know about. This includes the importance of medications, screenings, tests and procedures that are often recommended by practitioners for pregnant women.

Medications

There are some medications that you should be taking while you're pregnant and some medications that you should avoid for the safety of you and your baby. During your pregnancy, it is important not to take any medications unless first discussing them with your practitioner. This is true even for medications that you are currently taking. You should advise your practitioner of all medications you are currently taking, so he/she can help you determine which ones are safe for you to continue taking now that you know you are pregnant.

Unfortunately, it is hard to tell what is safe and not safe during pregnancy, even for a physician. This is because there is constant research about medications and their safety during pregnancy, causing the lists of safe and not-safe medications to change almost daily.

With that said, there are medications that you may need that are essential to your health. The only thing to consider is how will this affect your unborn child. Talking with a physician may provide some assistance, although not all are up-to-date on medications that have negative impacts on pregnancy.

For a more complete list of medications, feel free to contact your local March of Dimes office, contact the FDA or ask the pharmacist. Typically, these three resources will have the most up-to-date information regarding medication use during pregnancy.

Screening Tests

There are a wide variety of tests available to pregnant women. Some are specifically for those who are considered a high risk, are of a certain age when they become pregnant, or have a family history of certain medical conditions. Others are routine tests that are recommended for all pregnant women. Here you will find information on what tests there are, when and why they are conducted and what the risks associated with each are.

First Trimester Screenings

During your first trimester, some practitioners may recommend that you have a screening done for Down syndrome, to determine whether or not your baby may have this medical condition. This is conducted through an ultrasound, somewhere between weeks 10 and 14. During the ultrasound, the practitioner is looking for excess fluid around the neck of the fetus.

In conjunction with the ultrasound, a blood test is also involved, wherein your physician is looking for high levels of plasma protein A and hCG. Both of these are hormones produced by the fetus that are passed through the mother's bloodstream. If the results of this ultrasound are abnormal, then the practitioner would typically recommend a test known as amniocentesis.

Second Trimester Screening

During the second trimester a triple blood screen can be conducted to determine the risk of your baby having Down syndrome. The blood test is simple and is used to measure the amounts of three different hormones that are produced by the fetus and passed through the mother's bloodstream. The hormones are alpha-fetoprotein, hCG and estriol.

When the MSAFP test is conducted around the 15th and 18th weeks, abnormally high levels may be an indicator of spina bifida, while abnormally low levels may suggest and increased risk for Down syndrome. This does not mean that your baby will for sure have a birth defect, this is just an indicator that this is a possibility.

In fact, only one or two women, out of fifty, who have abnormal levels during these screenings will have a baby with birth defects. The other forty-eight may find that the levels were off due to a multiple birth, such as twins, the due date was calculated incorrectly or the results were just incorrect. In the event a followup ultrasound finds only one fetus and that the child is still in line with the due date, an amniocentesis is recommended.

Ultrasound

Ultrasound has made diagnosing pregnancy and issues with pregnancy a lot less complicated. Physicians also use ultrasounds in order to help you determine whether or not you are having a boy or a girl. Ultrasounds can be used at various times during pregnancy and for various reasons.

There are different levels of ultrasound used during pregnancy. A level one ultrasound is used to diagnose pregnancy and determine your due date. Typically this is conducted somewhere around the 12th week of pregnancy. A level two ultrasound is used during the 18th and 22nd weeks for diagnosing abnormalities with the pregnancy.

This may include determining the cause of bleeding you may be experiencing, locating an IUD that was in place when your baby was conceived and locating a fetus before other tests, such as a CVS and amniocentesis, are performed.

Further, an ultrasound during these weeks can be used to determine why a baby's heartbeat that was heard in the past using a Doppler is no longer able to be heard and also to determine why a mother may no longer be feeling movement.

In addition, an ultrasound can determine whether or not you are having more than one baby, such as twins or triplets and make sure there is an adequate amount of amniotic fluid for the baby. As you attend prenatal visits with your practitioner, they will measure the size of your uterus and if there are any abnormal growth patterns, an ultrasound may be used to determine the cause of abnormal growth.

Ultrasounds can also be used to detect cervical changes that could indicate going into labor prior to your due date, identify the location, maturity, size and/or abnormalities of the placenta and evaluate the condition of the fetus by monitoring fetal activity.

When it comes to delivery, an ultrasound can be used to make sure there the fetus is not in the breech position or any other abnormal position prior to making its way into the world. It can also be used to verify that the umbilical cord is not in a position that could cause complications during delivery.

It is important to understand that your practitioner may recommend an ultrasound at any time during pregnancy for a variety of reasons and it is really nothing to panic about. He/she will explain the reason they want to perform an ultrasound and let you know if there is anything you need to be concerned about.

There are two different ways a pregnancy ultrasound can be performed – abdominally and vaginally. There are times, however, when your practitioner may use both ways to find what they are looking for. As your uterus grows, the fetus does as well, often blocking the view of what your practitioner may be looking for.

Either way, the procedure does not last long, anywhere from 5-30 minutes, and are virtually painless. However, you will feel as though you need to urinate, because it is likely your practitioner will require a full bladder, particularly for the first trimester abdominal ultrasound.

You will be required to lay on your back for either procedure. During the abdominal ultrasound, your belly will need to be exposed and then they will place a gel on your abdomen, and push around a transducer. For a vaginal ultrasound, there is a different transducer that is inserted into the vagina.

With both procedures, the transducer records echoes of the sound waves as they bounce off various parts of both the mother and the fetus. These sound waves are translated into visual pictures. Often, the technician conducting the exam will point out various parts, such as the face, the arms, the legs, fingers and toes, as well as the heartbeat and spine. They will be able to take 'pictures' of your baby and print them out for you as well.

When it comes to the safety of an ultrasound, a lot of research has been conducted on the subject. To this day, there is no evidence that an ultrasound poses any risk to the mother or the fetus when used during pregnancy. However, practitioners still try to limit the number of ultrasounds conducted and only use them for valid reasons.

CVS (Chorionic Villus Sampling) Diagnostic Test

A Chorionic Villus Sampling or CVS test is another diagnostic test that can be used to provide reassurance during early pregnancy. The CVS test is typically performed in the first trimester and is used to diagnose birth defects, complications and genetic defects that may adversely affect your baby.

Although there is ongoing research to help increase the use of the CVS to detect more than 3,000 disorders related to defective genes and chromosomes, it is currently used to detect disorders, such as Tay-Sachs, some types of cystic fibrosis, sickle-cell anemia and Down syndrome. Typically, the test is conducted only when there is a family history of the disease or a parent is a known carrier.

The CVS test cannot, however, diagnose neural tube defects for other anatomical defects. If the CVS is a chosen diagnostic test, it would be conducted somewhere between the 10th and 13th weeks of pregnancy and is almost always performed in a hospital.

Depending on where the placenta is resting, the sample used for testing is taken through the vagina and the cervix. There are some cases where a needle can be inserted through the abdominal wall. Unfortunately, either method can range from slightly uncomfortable to very painful.

The test results for the CVS are usually available in about three to five days. When it comes to safety, there is some risk associated with the CVS testing, slightly more than the risks with amniocentesis. This includes an increased risk for miscarriage or limb deformities. With that said, however, most often the risk is typically associated with the experience of the technician performing the test. The more experienced an individual is, the less the risk of complications. It is recommended that you wait until you are at least 10 weeks along and you choose a center that has a high CVS success rate.

Amniocentesis Diagnostic Test

The amniocentesis is used to examine the amniotic fluid that carries your baby's cells and can be used to determine genetic makeup, the health condition of the fetus and the level of maturity. In most cases, amniocentesis is more than 99% accurate in determining whether or not your baby has Down syndrome.

There are specific conditions in which a physician recommends that this test be used to diagnose Down syndrome. This can range from the mother being more than 35 years old, having a child with Down syndrome, a close relative who has a neural tube defect, the mother has hemophilia or another X-linked genetic disorder and toxoplasmosis, for instance. There are others, but you should talk to your physician about the reasons why an amniocentesis may be appropriate for you.

If the decision is made to conduct amniocentesis, this procedure will be performed between the 16th and 18th weeks of your pregnancy. Studies have shown that risks associated with amniocentesis are highly increased when the test is conducted earlier than 14 weeks. In addition, amniocentesis can be used later in pregnancy, such as the last trimester, to ensure baby's lungs are working properly.

This test is conducted by use of an ultrasound so the technician can see what he/she is looking at. It is important that the fetus and the placenta are not disturbed during amniocentesis. A long needle is then inserted through the abdomen to withdraw a small amount of amniotic fluid from the uterus. Although the risk of poking the fetus is minimal due to the use of an ultrasound, there are still risks associated with amniocentesis.

There is not a lot of pain associated with amniocentesis, just some mild discomfort for a couple minutes to a few hours. You may also experience some mild cramping following the procedure. In very rare cases, you could see some light vaginal bleeding or have some amniotic fluid leak out. There are few women who have also obtained infections that have led to miscarriage. Therefore, amniocentesis is typically only used when the benefit of the results outweighs the risk of complication from the procedure.

What It All Means

These tests are not meant to scare you or create panic when your physician says them. They are not required and you should take time to decide before having them conducted. If you do choose to have any of these tests, you will really only find out what disorders or health conditions your baby may have.

The issue many women have with these types of tests is that it will not change how they feel about their baby, so they don't bother putting themselves or the child at risk for complications. They would prefer to wait until delivery day to learn all about their baby!

Talk with your doctor about the tests, the reasons why he/she has suggested them and determine together when the benefit outweighs the risks. Only then can you and your partner decide what's best for your family.

Chapter 4 – Food & Pregnancy – What's Right & Wrong

When you become pregnant, one of the first things you may notice is an increase in your eating habits. While you are now eating for two, this does not mean that you should eat double the amount. This actually means that you need to be careful of the foods you choose and ensure proper amounts of nutrition for your benefit and the benefit of your unborn baby.

Following the pregnancy diet is the simplest way to make sure both you and your baby will receive the nutritional components of food. This doesn't mean, however, that you can't send your partner for ice cream at eleven o'clock at night, it just means you shouldn't eat the whole gallon!

Prenatal Vitamins

As was mentioned earlier, getting an appointment with your practitioner as soon as possible is highly recommended. However, in the event that they cannot get you in for a few days or weeks, you need to ask when you call about prenatal vitamins. Although not a food group, prenatal vitamins help supplement your body by providing important vitamins and minerals that you may not adequately receive through food alone.

There are a variety of different types, from prescription brands to over-the-counter brands of prenatal vitamins. Your practitioner will decide which type you should take, how many, how often and when to start taking them, which is usually immediately.

Prenatal vitamins are the most important part of a pregnant woman's day. Prenatal vitamins are a specially designed vitamin for pregnant women and include all of the nutrients for the mother and the baby that are not typically consumed through food.

With that said, there are no standards set by the FDA or any other organization, to determine what must be in a prenatal vitamin. Typically, however, your practitioner will choose what they think is best for your specific health needs. If you choose an over-the-counter prenatal vitamin, it is important that you make sure an adequate amount of the right vitamins and minerals are in the supplement.

What you typically find in a prenatal vitamin is vitamin A, folic acid, calcium, iron, vitamin C, zinc, copper, vitamin B6, vitamin D, vitamin E, thiamin, riboflavin, niacin and vitamin B12. Each one provides some type of benefit for both the mother and the baby.

Your prenatal vitamin should contain 4,000 IU, or less, of vitamin A, as any more than 10,000 IU of vitamin A could be toxic. You should also be taking 250 mcg of calcium, 30 mg of iron, 80 mg of vitamin C, 15 mg zinc, 2 mg copper, 2 mg vitamin B6 and not more than 400 IU of vitamin D. The amounts of other minerals are quite small, but are provided in almost all prenatal vitamins.

It is important that you take your prenatal vitamins as directed by your practitioner or according to what the label says. Typically, you will take one in the morning and one in the evening, if it is an AM/PM vitamin or one per day, usually in the morning, if it is a one-a-day prenatal vitamin.

Further, it is important that you understand that taking a prenatal vitamin, no matter how much vitamins and minerals are in it, it should not replace a balanced, healthy diet. These vitamins are meant to be a supplement to your actual diet, ensuring that you are getting everything you and your baby need during pregnancy. You will learn about the different foods you should eat during pregnancy in a later chapter.

Benefits Of Pregnancy Diet

It is important that you understand why you need to eat the foods you do during pregnancy. That way, maybe you'll stick to the pregnancy diet a little more closely, because you know how important the benefits of the nutritious foods are.

First and foremost, eating healthy meals three times a day can increase the odds that your baby will be healthy. A nutritionally balanced diet can help ensure a healthy birthweight, improve fetal brain development and reduce the risk of some birth defects. Further, by starting your baby on nutritious foods in the womb, he/she will likely become a healthier adult later in life.

Eating a nutritionally balanced diet while pregnant provides other benefits for both you and your baby. You are more likely to have a safe, healthy pregnancy and possibly avoid complications, such as pre-eclampsia and anemia. Both of these conditions are more prominent in women who eat non-nutritious foods during pregnancy.

There is also the chance that eating healthier can reduce the occurrence of morning sickness, prevent fatigue, constipation and many other negative side effects of being pregnant. There has been research that healthy eating during pregnancy can become a mood booster, providing you with emotional stability and prevent mood swings.

A well-balanced diet during pregnancy has also been associated with on-time deliveries. This means that the healthier you and your baby are during pregnancy, the less of a risk for having a pre-term delivery. Furthermore, eating healthy can increase the recovery time for you post-partum, this includes losing 'baby weight'. Because you eat nutritious meals three times a day, you are less likely to gain too much weight at an increased pace during pregnancy. Therefore, following pregnancy, you are more likely to be able to shed those unwanted pounds.

Unfortunately, changing eating habits when you are pregnant is not an easy task. Dieting is a challenge for most women when they aren't pregnant. Add the increased occurrences of food cravings and eating for two and it's a whole other ball game. With that said, sticking to a pregnancy diet will take determination and hard work, but will definitely be worth it in the end.

Rules Of Healthy Pregnancy Eating

In order to stick to the pregnancy diet, there are a few basic rules you need to follow. These rules are designed to give you information about how much and how often you should and should not eat certain foods.

Each Bite Is Important

It is important that you pay attention to every bite you take. Each time you take a bite, think to yourself, "Is this bite of food going to benefit my baby?" If it is a healthy food that provides benefit to your baby – and you – then eat it. If you realize that maybe it's not so healthy of a food, try and find something that's a little better for you. With that said, there should be a bite or two that is purely meant to please your taste buds.

Understanding Calories

You should also understand that not all calories are created equal. You should select foods that have quality calories and not worry so much about the number. For instance, it is important that you choose a whole-grain raisin muffin that is 200 calories as opposed to a 200-calorie doughnut. While they have the same number of calories, the whole-grain raisin muffin provides you with nutrition. Another comparison – 100 calories of potato chips is completely different than a 100-calorie baked potato. The doughnut and chips provide you with calories while the muffin and baked potato have ingredients that will fill you up, leave you satisfied and provide vitamins and minerals essential to both you and your baby.

Eating efficiently is another rule you need to follow. What this means is that you the calories you take in have nutritional benefit, but also are important components of your diet. For instance, when it comes to calcium, you need quite a bit, however, you should not eat 1 ½ cups of ice cream that contains 450 calories to do this. Instead, choosing non-fat yogurt will give you the calcium you need, but only makes up for about 100 calories. The same goes for protein. While a 750 calories peanut butter sandwich with six tablespoons of peanut butter – who can eat that anyways – contains 25% of your needed protein, you would benefit more from a turkey burger, containing the same amount of protein and only 250 calories! Choose your calories wisely!

Starvation No – Regular Eating Yes

Just as you would never consider starving yourself, you should never starve your growing baby. Your baby needs regular nourishment at regular intervals. Although you may not feel hungry, your baby certainly is. Therefore, eating several small meals a day – and not skipping any – is the best way to providing nutrition to your baby. Research has found that expectant mothers who eat three regular meals plus to healthy snacks are less likely to have pre-term deliveries, meaning their babies are carried to full term.

Eat Good Carbohydrates Not Bad

One of the most difficult food groups to get a grasp on is carbohydrates. While you don't want to gain a lot of excess weight during pregnancy, cutting out carbohydrates is not necessarily the way to do it. You need the nutrition that 'good carbohydrates' can provide. For instance, a baked potato or whole-grain breads and cereals all have carbohydrates, but provide nutritional benefit. Also, fruits and vegetables naturally contain carbohydrates, but these should definitely be included in your pregnancy diet. Fruits that have skins on them, such as apples, as well as vegetables, such as potatoes, can provide you with B vitamins, minerals, protein and fiber, all of which are essential to a healthy pregnancy.

Foods that contain lots of fiber, such as fruits and vegetables, help you feel full and are not fattening, so they help you control your pregnancy weight gain. Further, they can diminish feelings of nausea and keep you from becoming constipated. It is best, however, that you choose fresh fruits and vegetables over those that are canned or frozen, as they tend to contain excess sugars. In addition, avoid refined grains by choosing whole grain foods, as these only provide you with non-nutritional carbohydrates, thus making them 'bad carbohydrates'.

Sweets

Calories that come from sweets are considered empty calories. Although these are okay once in a while, these types of calories add up quickly, taking away room for nutritional foods. Aside from leading to excessive weight gain, sugary foods can lead to tooth decay, heart disease, diabetes and colon cancer – none of which you want.

Unfortunately, sugar tends to find its way into a lot of different foods, by using a variety of types of sugar. For instance, high fructose corn syrup and dehydrated can juice are two types of sugars you will likely find in juices, beverages and canned fruits. Although honey is found in many nutritional foods, it's not necessarily any more beneficial than the refined sugars.

As a general rule, you want to limit your sugar intake as much as possible. When you do have sugary foods, try to choose those that have natural sugars, such as fruits. When choosing added sugars, try to get some nutritional benefit out of the products as opposed to choosing unhealthy foods that have added sugars. One suggestion is drinking fruit juice, because although it does contain sugar, there are vitamins and minerals contained in the fruit juice as well, which are essential to your pregnancy diet. These foods do provide sweetness for your taste buds, but also offer some vitamins and minerals that help to balance out your pregnancy diet.

Fresh Is Better

When it comes to choosing healthier foods, always choose fresh over any other variety, such as canned, frozen and/or processed. Fruits and vegetables tend to lose a lot of the nutrients you should be receiving when they are processed and packaged. Further, the way you cook a food can take away nutritional benefits. It is best to try and eat your fruits and vegetables fresh and raw to get the maximum nutritional benefit from them.

Include The Family

There is no reason you should be on the pregnancy diet alone. In fact, inviting your family to join in on your new eating habits is beneficial for everyone. Not only will this help you keep yourself on track, but in general, eating a well-balanced diet helps reduce the risk of you or your family members from developing a wide variety of health conditions later in life.

Further, having allies along for the ride can help you eliminate bad habits. This includes eating unhealthy foods, consuming alcohol, using tobacco products and/or illegal substances. If you take everyone around you on the pregnancy diet, you will be less likely to fail, ensuring a safe, healthy pregnancy for both you and your baby.

Allow Yourself To Cheat

You read earlier that it is okay to have a bite or two that isn't necessarily nutritious. It is okay to give into a food craving now and again, without feeling guilty about it, at least once a day. This doesn't mean that you should eat a gallon of ice cream. Choose frozen yogurt – similar to ice cream but provides nutritional benefit. You can also indulge yourself in one mildly unhealthy item per week, such as a fast food burger. Further, it's okay to have one completely unhealthy item that does nothing more than satisfy that craving you just can't seem to let go of. This could be a hot fudge sundae, a candy bar or a doughnut – anything you choose.

The important part about being on the pregnancy diet is that you do these things in moderation. Don't eat an entire bag of mini candy bars or a dozen of glazed doughnuts, but don't limit yourself completely either, as this can result in a complete failure of the pregnancy diet and unhealthy binge eating. Stay focused and allow yourself something now and then that just satisfies your taste buds and nothing more.

What Foods To Eat & How Much

Now that you know the basic rules of eating while pregnant, it is time to get a little more specific. In this section you will discover how many calories you should be consuming, as well as how much of eat food group is important per day. This includes protein, foods that contain vitamin C, calcium intake, how many servings of fruits and vegetables you need, the amount of whole grains you should incorporate, and the number of servings of iron-rich foods you need. Further, you will learn how much fat is okay to consume, how much salt and how much fluid you need per day.

Calories

When it comes to calories, just because you are eating for two doesn't mean you get to double the suggested caloric intake for one. In fact, a growing fetus really only needs about 300 calories per day, meaning you only need to add 300 calories per day, if you are of average weight, to keep your baby satisfied. However, during the first trimester, you actually need less than 300 calories per day added to your diet. That is, unless you are trying to make up for being underweight. As a general rule, if you are unsure about the exact number of calories you should be eating per day during each trimester, ask your practitioner what they suggest.

Protein

Protein is the building block of human cells, and therefore very essential in creating a human being – your growing baby. It is essential that you have three servings of lean protein per day, or about 60-70 grams. Although this may seem like a lot, you probably consume that already without even realizing it. However, now that you are pregnant, it is important that you keep track of what you are eating and how much, including protein.

Choose from tuna, skinless chicken breasts and turkey, lean beef, lamb, and pork for meat options. You can also choose products such as eggs (2 whole eggs), low-fat milk, tofu and/or vegetarian proteins. Make sure you are paying attention to the protein that is contained in high calcium foods as well, such as cottage cheese – this counts!

Vitamin C Foods

Vitamin C is essential in tissue repair, healing and other metabolic processes for both you and your baby. Vitamin C aids in the growth and development of strong bones and healthy teeth for your baby. It is important that you eat many foods that contain vitamin C each day. It is recommended that you eat these foods fresh and raw, as the vitamin is easily destroyed from cooking and air exposure.

Fruits that contain high amounts of vitamin C include grapefruits, oranges, mangoes, papayas, cantaloupe and strawberries. Vegetables that are high in vitamin C are broccoli, tomatoes, cauliflower, kale and raw cabbage.

Calcium

You need approximately 1,200 milligrams of calcium per day while you are pregnant. This helps provide your baby with a means to develop strong bones, healthy teeth and muscles. Calcium also helps increase heart and nerve development, conduce productive enzyme activity and aids in blood clotting.

However, calcium is not just for your baby – you need it too. If you are not consuming adequate amounts of calcium, your baby will steal yours. This leads to an increased risk of developing osteoporosis as you get older. It is very important that you get the suggested amount of calcium each day.

If milk is really not your thing, however, you need to be aware of other ways of getting the right amounts of calcium. Cottage cheese, cheddar, American and Swiss cheese all provide calcium, as does calcium-fortified orange juice, sesame seeds, tofu, broccoli, collard greens, kale and corn tortillas, to name a few. In addition, a variety of different fish can provide calcium, as long as they are prepared with the bones. This includes Pacific mackerel, salmon and sardines.

In the event you are unable to drink milk products, meaning you are lactose intolerant, you may want to consider speaking with your physician about a calcium supplement. It may be the only way you can get your proper calcium intake.

Fruits & Vegetables

There are two different categories when it comes to fruits and vegetables. The first category is green leafy and yellow vegetables combined with yellow fruits. The second category is all other fresh, raw fruits and vegetables.

For category one, it is important that you have at least three servings per day. The green leafy vegetables and yellow fruits and vegetables provide vitamin A, which is very important to cell growth for your baby. It also aids in developing bones, eyes and healthy skin, and has been associated with reducing the risk of developing cancer.

The green leafy vegetables and yellow fruits and vegetables also provide a long list of many other vitamins and minerals that are essential in fighting disease and preventing constipation, as they contain high amounts of fiber.

These foods include – cantaloupe, apricots (fresh or dried), yellow peaches, persimmon, canned unsweetened pumpkin, beet greens, raw carrots, winter squash and sweet potatoes, to name a few.

The second category – the other fruits and vegetables – are important to pregnancy, in that they provide magnesium and potassium, boron, phytochemicals and antioxidants. You can choose from just about any fruits and vegetables you can think of, such as bananas, apples, blueberries, grapes, bean sprouts, mushrooms, green beans, zucchini and potatoes, to name a few.

Whole Grains & Legumes

You need to have about six or seven servings of whole grains and/or legumes per day. This includes whole wheat, oats, rye, barley, corn, rice, peas, beans and peanuts. This category provides you with all sorts of nutrients, including various B vitamins that are essential for almost every part of your baby's development.

Further, these foods help you incorporate other aspects of the pregnancy diet, such as iron-rich foods and carbohydrates – the good variety. You can utilize whole grains almost anywhere when cooking, such as a pecan and whole grain breadcrumb breading for fish or chicken. You can also substitute rolled barley for recipes that call for oatmeal. These are great ways for incorporating whole grains and legumes into your diet.

Iron-Rich Foods

Iron is essential for developing and maintaining the baby's blood supply and for keeping you blood supply adequate. Further, when you are eating iron-rich foods, try to do it simultaneously with consuming foods that contain vitamin C, as it helps increase the absorption of iron by your body.

Foods that are rich in iron include lean cuts of beef, cooked oysters (don't eat raw ones), sardines, potatoes in the skin, pumpkin, spinach, green peas, chickpeas, lentils and other beans, soybeans and soybean products such as tofu and dried fruits, to name a few. Be sure to include as many of these types of foods as possible in your diet.

Fats

It is essential to include fat in your diet during pregnancy. In fact, 30% of the calories you consume while pregnant should be from fat. You need about four full servings of fat per day. This means that if you weigh about 125 pounds you would typically need about 2,100 calories per day, 630 of which should come from fat.

However, you should know that 630 calories of fat quickly adds up, as it only takes 70 grams of fat to reach this amount. You need to choose good fats, such as those that provide other nutritional benefits. This includes Swiss, provolone, mozzarella and cheddar cheeses, as well as sour cream, whole milk, cream cheese, peanut butter, ice cream, avocados, lean chicken or meat. When cooking, you can incorporate healthy fats and oils, such as vegetable oil, preferably olive oil, canola oil or walnut oil, butter, mayonnaise and salad dressing.

It is important, however, that you keep track of how much fat you are consuming. Too much fat could lead to excess weight gain for you and your baby. Balancing everything out is the key to a health pregnancy diet.

Salt

Salt can add flavor to your foods, but you need to be careful when consuming this seasoning. This means that you should not eat an entire bag of salted potato chips or a whole jar of pickles, both of which contain a lot of sodium. However, sodium depravation cause pose negative risk factors to your baby. It is important that you do have sodium in your diet, but instead of cooking with it, add just a little at the table. This helps you monitor your sodium intake. One last note – choose iodized salt, unless instructed by your practitioner, as this can help reach increase the levels of iodine in your body which is essential to pregnancy.

Fluids

Not enough can be said about the importance of fluid intake for any individual. However, this is even more important for an expectant mother. You need to remember that you are drinking for two now, and really be sure that you are getting adequate amounts of fluid, particularly water. You should be drinking about eight 8-ounce glasses of fluid per day.

Remember that most of the body of the baby inside you is comprised of water, much like yours. Fluid can help keep you skin soft, reduce the risk of constipation, remove toxins and waste products from your body and reduce swelling and the risk for developing urinary tract infections.

If you are retaining a lot of fluid, it is actually better for you to drink more. This is because, surprising as it may be, extra fluids can help flush out unnecessary build-ups of fluids. Although it is recommended that most of your fluid be from water, you can count other beverages as part of your fluid intake. This includes fruit and vegetables juices, soup, milk, decaffeinated tea and/or coffee and sparkling or flavored water.

You should avoid, however, drinking your calories. This means that if you are choosing to drink fluids other than water, that they be low-calorie beverages as opposed to high-calorie beverages. When it comes to soda, you can have some as long as it is caffeine and sugar free, but it still needs to be limited. It is also important that you do not drink right before eating, as this can make you feel full and not wanting to eat the foods that provide the nutrition you and your baby need.

Lastly, it is recommended that you spread your fluid intake out over the entire day. Start with a glass in the morning and then have another before lunch. Next, have a glass of fluid with lunch, then sometime after, with your afternoon snack – you're at four already. Have another glass an hour or so before dinner, one with dinner and one with your evening snack – that makes seven. Now, all you need is another glass later in the evening before going to bed. It is not recommended, however, that you drink more than two glasses at one time.

Chapter 5 – The First Trimester

Now that you know you are pregnant, understand a little bit about what you can and cannot eat, and some of the tests that will be conducted during pregnancy, it is time to take a trip through the first trimester, or first 13 weeks. This chapter will provide you with information, such as what the first prenatal visit will be like, how you may be feeling emotionally and physically as you progress through the first trimester, concerns about different symptoms and a variety of other topics that are all about getting you and your body used to being pregnant.

The First Prenatal Visit

As you know, one of the first things you should do is schedule a visit with your practitioner for a prenatal exam and checkup. As was already discussed, your practitioner will likely conduct a test to confirm that you are indeed pregnant. You will also need to discuss your complete medical history with your practitioner – leaving nothing out, even if it doesn't seem pertinent to you it may be important for you physician to know about.

There will also be a complete physical examination, which will consist of listening to your lungs and heart, a breast exam, determining a baseline blood pressure and taking note of your weight and height. Your practitioner may also check for any swelling and varicose veins, again serving as a baseline to compare with later examinations. There will also likely be an examination of your vaginal area, including your cervix and the size and shape of your pelvis, as this is where your baby will be exiting from. A Pap smear may also be conducted to look for signs of cervical cancer.

Also, there will be some tests either scheduled or conducting, depending on what your practitioner has available in his/her office. These tests are standard in pregnancy. They include a blood test to determine your blood type, whether you are Rh positive or negative, what your hCG levels are and to check for anemia. You will likely also need to have a urinalysis conducted to screen for glucose (to keep an eye on the development of gestational diabetes), check your protein levels, white blood cells, blood and screen for bacteria.

The blood test will also involve checking for disease, such as rubella, infections including syphilis, gonorrhea, hepatitis B, chlamydia and HIV. Depending on certain criteria, you may also be tested for cystic fibrosis, Tay-Sachs, sickle-cell anemia and other genetic diseases.

Month 1

During the first month, you will likely be noticing some physical and emotional changes with your body. Although you may stain lightly at the time your period is regularly due, you should not have any bleeding during this time. It is important that you discuss any bleeding you do experience with your practitioner right away, as this could be signs of complications.

You will also begin to become more exhausted, feel fatigue and sleepy, as there are a lot of internal changes taking place. As was mentioned earlier, you will feel the need to urinate frequently, may experience nausea with and/or without vomiting, heartburn, gas, bloating and indigestion. Pregnancy is often associated with food cravings, but you also may be experiencing food aversions. This means that even some of your favorite foods that you eat often you may not want anything to do with, including the smell.

One of the most significant changes you will notice physically is changes with your breasts. They may feel fuller, more tender, feel heavy and possibly tingly. You may even notice that the areola – the area surrounding your nipples – may become increasingly darker and the sweat glands may begin to look like very large goose bumps.

When it comes to emotions, they are comparable to a rollercoaster for most women. You will be very unstable, irritable, have mood swings, think irrationally, and often want to cry. In other words, it is okay to feel like an emotional basket case. You may also be experiencing feelings of joy, excitement and fear about having a baby.

Your bay is growing as well. By the end of the first month, you baby is a very tiny (smaller than a grain of rice), tadpole-like embryo. However, as tiny as your baby is, he/she will have already developed a head and mouth opening, a pumping heart, and a undeveloped brain. As of now, there are no arms or legs, but they will begin appearing soon.

Month 2

You've made it to month two of pregnancy and may have noticed some changes from last month to now. You will have another checkup to make sure you and your baby are progressing along fine. During this visit, you will have your weight and blood pressure measured, a urine sample – this will happen every month, so avoid going to the bathroom just before arriving – to check for sugar and protein levels and to make sure you are not dehydrated.

In addition, your practitioner will likely check for signs of swelling and varicose veins and compare those to last month. You should discuss any symptoms that you have experienced during the last month, especially mentioning any unusual symptoms. Also, make sure you have a list of questions ready for your practitioner, as once you get there you may forget something you wanted to ask about.

Physically, you probably are not feeling that much different now than you were a month ago. You will likely still be tired, have to go to the bathroom often, you may still be experiencing nausea and/or vomiting, heartburn, indigestion, gas and bloating. Differently, however, you may be slightly constipated and while this is something you should mention to your practitioner, if you notice this beforehand, try and increase your fiber intake a little at a time, as this can help with constipation.

In addition to the food cravings and aversions and breast changes from last month, you may notice a few other new symptoms. This can include a whitish vaginal discharge known as leukorrhea and you may experience headaches, occasional dizziness or feeling faint, and you may begin to notice that your clothes aren't fitting as well, particularly around your breasts and abdomen. You will also notice, as you may have last month, veins popping up across your stomach and your breasts. This is perfectly normal and a sign that your body is progressing along through pregnancy appropriately. Emotionally, you are still experiencing the same types of feelings in month two, as you did in month one.

Just like last month, your baby is continually growing. If you could see him/her right now, you would start to see that they are looking more like a baby and less like an embryo. The tail is gone and by the end of month 2, the arms and legs are apparent, complete with fingers and toes. You would also be able to see eyes, ears, a nose and tongue. Although they still have a lot more developing to do, all of the major organs are present by month two as well. You will not notice it for many weeks, but your baby is constantly on the move and the placenta, the baby's support system, is rapidly being created.

Month 3

Month three is the last month of the first trimester. Following this month, you will be in the second trimester of your pregnancy and at the start of 14 weeks. However, for now, there are some things you need to be aware of. You will again have a visit to the practitioner, but this time it will be slightly different than previous checkups.

Your practitioner will, as he/she has in the past, check your weight and blood pressure and urine. What is different this month, is listening to the fetal heartbeat using a Doppler, which is a very exciting time. Your practitioner will likely feel the outside of your abdomen, checking for the size of the uterus and make sure that the size is parallel to what the calculated due date is. It is possible for due dates to change early in pregnancy, as you progress, but this is not often the case, especially if you knew the date of your last menstrual period.

The height of the fundus, meaning the top of the uterus, will be measured. This is important, as by the time you reach near your due date, the fundus will have reached your bellybutton. As long as your baby is growing and developing on schedule, your fundus should be a certain length at each visit, or around about a certain length. Lastly, your practitioner will check to see how you are doing when it comes to swelling and varicose veins, again referring to notes about previous visits regarding the same.

Physically, you will not experience many changes from the previous two months, in that you will still be tired, have to urinate often and may still be experiencing nausea and vomiting as well as constipation. Everything else will be the same, as well, such as heartburn, food aversions and cravings, breast changes, headaches and dizziness, and the tightening of clothing.

One thing you may notice that hasn't really changed in prior months, but is changing now, is your appetite. You will likely begin feeling hungry a lot more often than you have in the past. This is because your baby is growing and needs more nutrients, thereby taking them from you, stealing your food and making you hungrier more often.

Chapter 6 – The Second Trimester

You have now reached the beginning of your second trimester, which for most women is typically the most comfortable trimester of the three. While the first brings on changes and morning sickness and the third you really get uncomfortable as the baby is starting to run out of room, the second trimester seems to fit everyone a little better.

During this stage of pregnancy, you will still continue to have monthly visits with your practitioner and you may notice some different physical and emotional changes and most likely, if you haven't already, you will begin to show – meaning others may notice that you are pregnant, if they haven't already. Here's a look – month by month – of your second trimester of pregnancy.

Month 4

During your visit to the practitioner in month four you will experience the same round of tests – urine, weight and blood pressure and listening to the fetal heartbeat. Your practitioner will also feel the outside of your abdomen, determining the size of your uterus, the height of the fundus will be measured again and you will be checked for swelling and varicose veins, again comparing to past notations regarding these conditions. You should also continue to discuss any symptoms you are experiencing and ask any questions you have about your pregnancy.

Physically, you will begin to notice some changes, most of which are for the good. Although you will still be fatigued, this may decrease to some degree, and you might make it through the day without desperately needing a nap. However, there is no rule that says you cannot take a nap if you have the time, as long as you are getting adequate sleep at night – about 7-8 hours per night.

Fortunately, the need to urinate every five minutes will likely decrease by the fourth month as well and for those who experienced 'morning sickness' it is likely to subside. On the other hand, there are women who can continue to feel nausea and occasionally vomit, while for others, the fourth month could be the start of 'morning sickness'.

Constipation often continues through the entire time you are pregnant, and you should not be alarmed, but again, you may need to increase your fiber intake to help aide in regular bowel movements. The same goes for heartburn, indigestion, gas, bloating, headaches and dizziness.

In addition, you will continue to feel and see your breasts becoming larger, but could benefit from a decrease in the tenderness felt in the first trimester. However, the fourth month does bring some new physical symptoms that you could experience.

This includes nasal congestion accompanied by nosebleeds and ear stuffiness at times, as well as, blood when brushing your teeth from your gums bleeding and again, an increase in your appetite will still be apparent.

You may begin to notice swelling of your extremities, hands and feet in particularly, and maybe even your ankles and face on occasion. You may begin to notice the development of varicose veins and/or hemorrhoids.

While all these seem quite uncomfortable, you have one exciting physical symptom to look forward to toward the end of the fourth month – fetal movement. This is particularly the case with women who are thinner prior to becoming pregnant and those who are expecting their first child. For others, this may not happen for another month or so.

Emotionally, you continue to be a rollercoaster. You will experience instability and mood swings, parallel to your behavior during PMS. You may, however, begin to feel apprehensive about the way you are looking, feeling fat rather than pregnant. It is important however, to remember that pregnancy is a beautiful thing and it's okay not to fit in your normal clothes.

This too, is a concern for many women, wherein they don't fit in their regular clothes anymore, but just are not ready to wear maternity clothing either. This can often cause frustration and anxiety about finding things to wear from day to day.

You may also be feeling a little scatter-brained, forgetful and feel like you are having trouble concentrating. Do not fret, however, as these feelings are quite normal. Pregnancy does a lot to a body and it can take some time getting used to. It is still important to relax as much as you can, continue the rules of the pregnancy diet and make sure you are getting plenty of fluids.

As for your baby during month four, new changes are happening. Your baby is probably about five inches, give or take a few, which is a major increase from being the size of a rice grain only three months ago! He/she, however, probably only weighs about five ounces at this point as well and the body is growing faster than the head, so as to catch up and begin taking on more human-like features.

It is likely that at this point the fingerprints and toe prints have developed and temporary hair, known as lanugo, has begun to appear on the body. Your baby may be able to suck his/her thumb, swallow amniotic fluid and secrete it as urine and begin practicing breathing techniques.

Also during the fourth month, the placenta has become fully functional and can provide the baby with nourishment and oxygen. If your baby is a girl, she will have developed a uterus and ovaries equipped with primitive egg cells. The bones of your baby are becoming harder and he/she will begin moving his/her arms and legs, which is why you may begin feeling kicks.

Month 5

If you haven't already felt them, you will most likely begin feeling the baby 'kick' as he/she moves around the uterus and your belly will become rounder – welcome to month five of pregnancy.

You will again have an appointment with your practitioner, wherein he/she will conduct the usual tests – weight and blood pressure, urine, measure the uterus by feeling on the outside of your abdomen, measure the height of the fundus and check for swelling of the feet and hands. You will also be able to hear the baby's heartbeat during your visit. Again, you should discuss any unusual symptoms and ask any questions that have come about since last month about your pregnancy.

Physically, you will be feeling fetal movement by this point, which is something very exciting, as it really makes it hit home that you having a little human being growing inside your uterus. It really, truly is an amazing feeling.

You will continue to experience the same symptoms as you had in the fourth month, from constipation and heartburn to gas and bloating, headaches and dizziness. You may still experience nasal congestion, nosebleeds and/or ear stuffiness, as well as bleeding gums.

However, a few things are different, which will continue to be the trend until you reach delivery. You may begin to feeling some aches in your lower abdomen as a result of your muscles stretching to accommodate the growing uterus as your baby grows. You may begin to have a very hearty appetite, and can experience leg cramps and swelling of the hands, feet and ankles.

Do not be too concerned if you start to notice that your heart rate (pulse) is slightly higher than normal, or if the color of your skin, particularly around your face and abdomen change slightly. These are all signs and symptoms associated with pregnancy. A benefit, however, that you may notice during the fifth month is that orgasms may be easier to achieve, which is most likely attributed to swelling and pushing down of your vaginal cavity making it easier for your partner to hit 'the spot'.

Unfortunately, you may begin to feel the aches and pains in your back that are caused from the excess weight you are carrying in the front and you may begin to notice that your bellybutton is starting to protrude from its original position.

Emotionally, you may begin to gain a sense of reality that you are pregnant, but you will likely experience less mood swings, or at least less severe mood swings. However, it is still possible to experience weepiness, irritability and a feeling of being absentminded.

As your belly grows, you can be sure that the reason is because your baby is growing too. In fact, during month five there are some major changes happening inside your uterus. Your baby is typically somewhere between seven and nine inches in length and could weigh as much as a pound. The muscles are becoming stronger, nerve networks are expanding and the skeleton continues to harden.

Because of these three events, it is likely that your baby is becoming more active, performing somersaults (literally) and flipping all around your uterus. This is why you will most likely begin feeling the sensations of kicking and poking from inside your stomach. In addition, your baby's ears are fully developed now and he/she can begin hearing and recognizing sounds. Odd as it may seem, your baby will also have periods of being awake and periods of being asleep – unfortunately these events do not always coincide with your sleeping patterns.

Because your baby is continually growing and figuring out new features of himself/herself, they have the ability to make different faces, including frowns and grimaces, which can make for adorable ultrasound photos. What makes these faces even more realistic, is the development of eyebrows and head hair during month five.

Your baby's skin is also beginning to change and has become wrinkly, pink, translucent and covered in a vernix, which is a greasy substance that helps protect the baby from amniotic fluid and helps make the baby slippery, which makes delivery more easy. If your baby is a boy, his testicles will drop down from the abdominal cavity into the scrotum.

During the fifth month, if you haven't been counting, you will come across 18-20 weeks, wherein your practitioner will likely schedule an ultrasound, which has more than one benefit. This ultrasound is considered routine and is just your practitioner's way of checking up on baby. Because sexual organs have developed for both boys and girls at this point, it is a way for parents to discover the sex of their baby – if they want to. Even if you do not want to know whether you are having a boy or girl, you will at least get to have a look-see at your little baby!

Month 6

Although there may be variations due to your practitioner's style and your personal needs, your six-month checkup will pretty much be business as usual – weight and blood pressure testing, urinalysis, to check for sugar, protein and adequate fluid intake, fetal heartbeat, height of fundus, size of uterus (from the outside), checking for swelling and discussing any symptoms you are experiencing or questions you may have.

Physically, you will definitely be noticing more and more movement coming from inside your uterus. You may also continue to have a whitish vaginal discharge, be constipated and feel minimal aches around the bottom side of your abdomen. You may or may not continue to experience any of the other symptoms you have been feeling – or may just be experiencing them for the first time.

This includes heartburn, gas, bloating, indigestion, headaches, dizziness, nasal congestion and nosebleeds, ear stuffiness and bleeding gums as well as a continue desire to eat. Some women still experience leg cramps and swelling, along with a backache.

However, as you progress through pregnancy, the list of symptoms continues to get much longer of things you may experience. This includes an itchy abdomen, continually protruding navel, enlarged breasts, skin color changes around the abdomen and face.

Emotionally, things are beginning to change a little as well. You may experience fewer mood swings, but at the same time you may be wondering if anybody will talk to you about anything aside from being pregnant for a change. You may continue to feel absentminded and start having anxiety about the upcoming delivery.

Your baby has grown quite a bit this last month and is probably over a foot long by now and weighs in at around two pounds. He/she is also continuing to be quite active and is actually becoming more coordinated and may have the ability to peddle his/her feet and push up against the wall of your uterus. The baby is developing his/her gripping muscles now and may use them to grab ahold of the umbilical cord. Fortunately, the umbilical cord is strong and made of spirals, which help keep it from knotting or twisting to where it would cut off the baby's lifeline.

Your baby's eyes are working, opening and closing, and he/she may even close them, or use his/her hands to protect them when a bright light is shone at your belly. This means that your baby is reactive to light. Amazingly, the vocal cords are in full working order, but your little one will not be exercising these for another couple months, when you hear the first cry at delivery. He/she may also hiccup quite often and shake the uterus, which you may or may not feel.

As you get closer to your due date – you have a ways to go from here – the risk of premature labor could be weighing on your mind. Although you would prefer to carry full term, in the event something happens that causes you to go into labor early, you should know that the probability of your child surviving with the help of intensive care is in your favor. This is because all major organs are functioning, although prematurely, and with a little help, he/she should be just fine.

Chapter 7 – The Third Trimester

You have successfully made it to your third – and final – trimester. Congratulations, you're almost ready to have your little bundle of joy come into the world.

Month 7

The seventh month, which encompasses weeks 28-31, brings some differences when it comes to your prenatal visit with your physician. Your weight and blood pressure will still be checked, as will your urine, the fetal heartbeat, the height of the fundus and swelling. When it comes to the uterus, your practitioner will feel the outside for the size and actually the position of the uterus this time. This is because your due date is fast approaching and he/she needs to make sure the baby is getting ready, as you are.

Depending on your practitioner's rules and style of practicing, you will likely be required to have a blood test, checking for anemia and what is called a glucose screening test. You practitioner may explain that the glucose screening test is to check for gestational diabetes, which you can read about in the Q&A section at the end of the book.

As far as the test goes, it's fairly simple. You will go to the lab, hospital or wherever your practitioner sends you about the 28th week. This is a standard test and is ordered for about 99% of pregnant women, even if they do not have diabetes or a risk for developing diabetes. What you will do is drink a very sweet – glucose – beverage, usually fruit flavored and then wait about an hour before having your blood drawn.

Once the test results are in, if you have elevated numbers, this may suggest that your body may not be producing enough insulin to process extra glucose in your system. If this is the case, you will be required to take a glucose tolerance test. For this test, you need to fast, meaning eating nothing or drinking nothing for a certain period of time. You will then need to drink another glucose beverage, although this one has a higher concentration of glucose, and then wait three hours before having your blood drawn. This is how gestational diabetes is diagnosed.

There are quite a few additions when it comes to physical symptoms. You will likely continue to experience what you have been for the last six months, but the seventh month brings new issues. You may start to notice that you feel short of breath, have difficulty sleeping and you may experience occasional Braxton Hicks contractions. These are typically painless, but your uterus will contract and then relax.

These Braxton Hicks contractions are a type of rehearsal for the real labor and delivery of your baby. If you have had a pregnancy prior to this one, you may feel these contractions earlier in pregnancy and they may also be slightly more painful. But for a first-timer they typically do not present until after the 20th week, although you probably haven't noticed them until now.

As you get closer to your due date, you may experience longer more frequent Braxton Hicks contractions, although you're not quite ready for delivery and these types of contractions are not sufficient for childbirth. They are, however, a precursor to the real thing and help with effacement and early dilation of the cervix. In a sense, Braxton Hicks are a type of warning sign that you are getting ready for delivery.

What happens during this time is that for about 15-30 seconds, although they can last up to a few minutes, your uterus contracts and then releases. Typically, it will begin at the top and you will feel it harden, then progress downward, releasing as it reaches the bottom of the uterus.

Even though Braxton Hicks are not true signs of labor, as you get closer to your due date, they may be harder to distinguish from the real thing. It is important that you describe, in detail, how these contractions are making you feel to your practitioner. He/she will be able to help you determine whether or not you are truly in labor or just experiencing Braxton Hicks contractions.

Another note – if you begin to experience them more often, up to four times per hour, it is important that you call your practitioner immediately. This is especially true if the contractions are associated with back pain, abdominal pain or pain in your pelvis, or if you have any increase in vaginal discharge or at an increased risk for premature labor.

Emotions are still in full force, although it's likely that the mood swings have dissipated and you are now experiencing excitement and joy. You may however, still feel slightly apprehensive about labor, delivery and becoming a mother, particularly if this is your first child. You may begin, if you haven't already, imagining what your baby will be like when he/she is born. You may still experience feelings of being absentminded and you could feel either bored with the pregnancy – ready to get it over with and meet your baby – or you may feel happy and content. This is particularly true in women who are getting plenty of rest, eating the right foods and are feeling physically energized.

As far as your baby goes this month, he/she is gaining weight at a very fast rate, probably weight three pounds, and growing fast too, around 16 inches long. If you could see your baby now, you will notice fat deposits developing under the skin and the Lanugo hair is starting to disappear.

In the meantime, your baby's head hair is rapidly growing, as are the eyebrows and eyelashes. Nails are now at the tips of the fingers and toes and the skin is pink and smooth – no longer translucent. If your baby is light-skinned, he/she will have blue eyes at this point, and if your baby is dark-skinned, he/she will have brown eyes. However, this does not necessarily determine the color of your baby's eyes. The true color typically does not develop until weeks or months after birth

Over the next few months your baby's brain will begin developing at a fast pace, also, and will continue over the first two years of life. The lungs are beginning to function, only they are still immature. A baby born during the seventh month, although premature, has a very good chance of survival.

Month 8

The eighth month – only one more to go before delivery – is pretty much standard when it comes to visits with your practitioner. However, now that you are 32 weeks pregnant, you may need to come in every two weeks, so that your progress can be monitored a little closer. When it comes to what your practitioner will do during the visits, it's pretty much the same as in the past. You will have your weight and blood pressure checked, your urine will be screened for sugar, protein and dehydration, the fetal heartbeat will be listened to and you will be checked for swelling in your hands and feet.

Again, the height of the fundus will be measured, as will the size and position of the fetus inside your uterus. By using their hands, it is possible that your practitioner can feel where your baby is, and get a rough estimate of their size by feeling on the outside of your abdomen. You should discuss any unusual symptoms, ask questions, and describe any symptoms of Braxton Hicks or other contractions.

During the eighth month, your practitioner may order a test for Group B strep sometime after the 35th week, but prior to the 37th week. This is a bacterium that can be found in the vaginas of women, even healthy women. If you are carrying these bacteria, it actually poses no harm to you, but can be passed to your baby during delivery and could pose a risk for developing a very serious infection.

You will show no signs or symptoms of having Group B strep, therefore testing for it is the only way it can be found. When it comes to Group B strep, it is better to be safe than sorry, to avoid causing infection or harm to your newborn. The test is fairly simple, much like a Pap smear, in which your vagina and rectum will be swabbed and then tested. If you do test positive, you will be given IV antibiotics during labor to protect your baby. If GBS is found in the urine, you will be given oral antibiotics during the last few weeks of pregnancy.

Not much changes physically, except for perhaps the size of your belly, during the eighth month. You may become slightly clumsy, as the weight of the fetus is affecting your balance and you may find it difficult to sleep, possibly because of the size of your abdomen. Your breasts will continue to become enlarged and you could possibly see colostrum leaking from your nipples. This is a premilk substance that develops for breastfeeding. There is a possibility that this will not actually occur until after delivery, but still something you should be aware of, so you do not panic.

Emotionally, you are probably ready to delivery your baby, may because of being uncomfortable or just due to pure excitement. However, you have a few weeks to go, so hang in there. You may still continue to feel apprehensive about various topics – becoming a mother, you and your baby's health and labor and delivery. Feeling this way is normal, nine months is a long time to think about something before it occurs. Unfortunately, you are likely to still be slightly absentminded, and eventually this will dissipate, though probably not immediately following birth or even when you get home, as you will likely be sleep deprived the first few months of your baby's life.

Your baby has likely reached a length of 18 to 20 inches and could be weighing about five to six pounds at this point. He/she will continue to gain about ½ ounce per day until delivery. Your baby is looking a lot less wrinkly, due to the increasing development of fat deposits filling in the body. Those cute and adorable creases around the wrists are likely formed by this point and if your baby is born with dimples, those will be apparent now also.

Your abdomen is now quite large, but unfortunately, the womb is becoming more and more crowded for your baby. You will not likely feel any gymnastics-like activity going on, but may feel as though feet and toes are jammed into your ribs. There is a possibility that your baby is just as uncomfortable as you are, as his/her home is getting much smaller. Vigorous kicking will likely have subsided, but you could feel more twisting, as the baby tries to move about.

Fortunately, they will not always be grabbing or kicking at your ribs, as your baby will experience periods of deep sleep, what is referred to as REM sleep, periods of quite resting, and periods where he/she seems to do nothing but squirm around.

Still, your baby's brain and lungs continue to develop, with lungs reaching near full working capacity, making it less scary to go into premature labor at this point. If premature labor does occur, do not worry, at this point, your baby has a very excellent chance of not only surviving, but being very healthy as well.

Month 9

You've reached the final four weeks of pregnancy – congratulations! As things come to an end you may feel like you should pack your bags and sleep at your practitioner's office, as you will be there very often – typically about once a week at least. The visit, though typically the same, does present with some difference, and you may notice quite a bit of changes in your body at this point. Here's a look at month nine on the pregnancy timeline.

Your weight and blood pressure will be tested as usual, although what you see on the scale and the blood pressure reading may be slightly different. In fact, weight gain at this point is typically very slow, if you gain any weight at all. As for your blood pressure, it is possible for it to be slightly higher than it has been in the past. Your urinalysis will be the same and you will be checked for swelling and varicose veins, as usual.

The height of the fundus will be measured and you will get to have a listen at the fetal heartbeat. When your practitioner is checking your fetus, by using his/her hands on the outside of your abdomen, they are checking for the position and size of the fetus, possibly providing a rough guess about the weight of your baby.

You will also have an internal examination that can help the practitioner determine whether or not your cervix has begun to thin out (effacement) or start to open (dilation). This may begin early and continue slowly as you progress through the next couple of weeks.

When it comes to fetal position, there are quite a few ways your baby could be lying – vertex, frank breech, footling and traverse. The majority of babies present in the vertex position, meaning head first, on the day of delivery. However, there are some babies that come out bottom first with legs up by their face, which is known as the frank breech position. Still, some may choose to come feet first, known as the footling position or are currently lying sideways in what is known as the traverse position.

Your practitioner may give you advice on how to help the baby turn, if he/she does not seem to be wanting to move. The most ideal position for your fetus during delivery is the vertex position. Although children can be born with minimal complications in the frank breech or footling position, it is quite difficult for both mother and baby, causing stress. For babies in the traverse position who do not turn, or to prevent complications from other positions, your practitioner may recommend you have a cesarean section – C-section, which will be discussed in detail in the labor and delivery chapter.

Take the time during these last few visits to obtain clarification on any questions you have related to labor and delivery. Your practitioner and you both need to know what the other is considering and thinking when it comes to how you want to go about childbirth. If you want to attempt a natural childbirth, meaning no medications, you need to clarify this with your physician, so he/she is aware of your wishes.

Physically, you will still experience the same symptoms you have dealt with over the last eight months, with some increased pain and discomfort due to the size of your abdomen and how your fetus moves. Fetal movement will continue to be felt, although smaller movements that can still be quite uncomfortable, as he/she is running out of room.

If you felt a shortness of breath in the past, you may get some relief in the ninth month. This is due to your baby dropping into position and taking pressure off of your upper body, including your lungs. However, when the baby drops you may feel an increase in the need to urinate, as he/she may now be pushing on your bladder again.

Braxton Hicks contractions may continue and become longer and more painful and you may have a rough time getting around, as you will become more clumsy, as the baby moves around and sets you off balance. You may begin to develop nesting syndrome, which means that you may alternate between periods of fatigue and excess energy, and you may either have an increased appetite or possibly no appetite at all.

Emotionally, you may be feeling relief at the thought of your pregnancy being almost over, but still impatient about the event, as you still have a few weeks. You may be irritable and oversensitive, particularly when people make comments like, "didn't you have that baby yet?', as they can be quite frustrating to hear. Take these comments and let them go in one ear and out the other, or just brush them off with a laugh, even though you'd really like to punch the individual who said it, thinking to yourself, why don't you carry this baby around for nine months!

It's okay to feel frustrated and anxious about being pregnant at this point. You have spent nine months carrying around another human being inside you and dealing with quite a lot of symptoms, aches and pains, even in a normal, healthy pregnancy. But don't worry, you will soon realize – in a few weeks – that everything you have gone through was worth it, as you will get to hold and kiss your newborn baby.

Speaking of which, your baby has grown some this month as well, and is preparing to make a move toward the exit sign at some point near the end of the month. Your baby will officially be a full term baby by week 38, although delivery at any point in the last month is considered safe in a normal pregnancy. Your baby has probably grown an additional two inches and put on about 2 ½ pounds and by the delivery day, your baby will be about 15% body fat.

As for your baby's current home, the umbilical cord has likely grown to be about two feet long and the placenta probably weighs in at an additional 1 ½ pounds. This is a plus, as not only will you lose the weight of your baby, but the next time you step on the scale, you will be an additional 1 ½ pounds lighter, just from delivering the placenta.

At some point during month nine, you will move into the labor and delivery stage of pregnancy and childbirth, which is discussed in the next chapter.

Chapter 8 – Childbirth – What You Need To Know

It's time to have a baby! There are a lot of different aspects to childbirth, from contractions, to methods of giving birth and the use of medications. Over the last nine months, you have prepared for this day and hopefully made it a point to discuss with your practitioner your wishes when it comes to labor and delivery.

If you chose an obstetrician, you will be having your baby in a hospital, in the maternity ward, which is designed specifically for women having babies and the initial care of your baby at birth. It is likely also, that a pediatrician will show up just as the baby is born to give him/her a checkup and run a few standard tests, such as determining the Apgar score, hearing and vision-type tests.

If you are using a midwife, you may be having your baby at home or in a birthing center, which you have probably discussed with your practitioner as well, over the last nine months. Either way, it is important that you relax, follow all instructions of your practitioner and enjoy yourself, because it is all worth it when you see those chubby cheeks, arms and legs, holding your baby for the first time.

It is important to understand that this chapter focuses on a vaginal delivery. If you are concerned about a cesarean section, please refer to the Q&A section provided in chapter ten.

Stage One – Labor

Childbirth has been divided, by Mother Nature originally and then by obstetrics, into three phases, early labor, active labor and transitional labor, which brings your cervix to a full dilation, in preparation for delivery of both your baby and your placenta. The time spent on labor and delivery can cover a wide range of times, varying from a few hours to a lot of hours, depending on whether or not this is your first delivery or not, and how quickly your cervix dilates.

If you are not progressing along, and your cervix is not opening, your practitioner may enlist the help of a pregnancy inducer known as Pitocin. In fact, some practitioners begin labor by using Pitocin to get things moving and if your water does not break on its own, they may do it for you, again to help increase the start of your cervix dilating.

Other than that, you may begin to notice the signs of labor on your own, such as contractions, your water breaking or the loss of your mucous plug, accompanied by a little bloody show. A mucous plug is a blog-like gelating barrier that has kept your cervix from opening prior to delivery. Sometimes, as labor begins, this can become dislodged and allow for effacement of your cervix. Many women do not experience the passing of a mucous plug and is not a reliable source or signal for labor starting. You may lose your mucous plug several weeks before labor begins, but it will allow for your cervix to begin opening.

If you do happen to have a small amount, what's known as a bloody show, this could be a more realistic indicator that labor is in progress, as this means that your cervix is starting to open to allow for the fetus to come through the canal. But unfortunately, until you have true contractions, this may take some time as well, but it is a good sign that things are getting started.

Phase One – Early Labor

The first phase of labor, also known as early or latent labor, is typically the longest phase of labor. Your cervix is beginning to thin out and will slowly dilate until it has become about 3 centimeters. While this does not seem like very much, it could take days or weeks to reach those 3 centimeters. Fortunately, during this time you will likely not have any contractions, or if you do they will often go unnoticed.

If you do have contractions during early labor, they typically last anywhere from 30-45 seconds, but are often shorter in length. On the pain scale, they are usually mild to moderate and can be regular, close to five minutes apart or irregular, more than 20 minutes apart. However, they can also occur at any interval in between.

Although contractions at an early phase typically do not become consistent, they will continue to get closer together. However, you may not even realize you are experiencing contracts. If you do notice them, and call your practitioner, you will likely be sent to the hospital, which brings phase one to an end and you will likely be entering into phase two – active labor.

During your time in early labor you may experience a wide variety of common symptoms associated with early labor. This can include backaches, either constant or just presenting with each contraction, cramping similar to menstrual cramps, indigestion, diarrhea and a warm sensation in your abdomen. You may also experience a bloody show, as was discussed in the beginning of the chapter.

If your water (amniotic membranes) rupture on their own, it is possible for this to occur during this phase. However, this mostly likely occurs later in labor, or as was already mentioned, by your practitioner artificially.

You may be an emotional wreck at this point, and experience feelings of excitement, fear, anxiety, uncertainty, anticipation and relief all at the same time. However, there are some women who breeze through this phase and continue to be relaxed and chatty about the situation.

Although you are experiencing a lot of emotions at once, it is best to try and relax. Calling the practitioner is not a necessity at this point, unless of course your water has broken or you have heavy vaginal bleeding, in which case you would need to go to the emergency room at the hospital, because labor is in full force.

If contractions come while you are asleep, waking you up, try and get as much rest as you can, the next several hours are going to be long enough, but can be made worse by a lack of sleep. If this phase begins during the day, try and go about your normal activities, making sure you are not too far from home or the hospital.

You can take a walk to help move labor along, or just sit and relax, maybe watch some TV or read a book. You could also make up one of your favorite meals and put it in the freezer for a quick dinner during post-partum recovery, as you likely won't have the energy or time – as your baby will be taking most of it – to cook at that point. If you haven't already, now is the time to pack your bags for the hospital. It is recommended that you don't pack anything tight-fitting, even though you are about to lose a lot of excess weight. Your body will be slightly swollen after labor and tight fitting close may irritate you. Make sure you have your soaps, shampoos, a comb, toothbrush and whatever you need to make you feel like you're at home. You will be spending a few nights, more if you are planning a C-section, in the hospital.

You should also let your spouse know what is happening, although there is no point in him rushing home right now. You still have a few hours, again, as long as your water didn't break and you aren't experiencing any vaginal bleeding.

It is also recommended that you try and make yourself as comfortable as possible. As long as your water hasn't broken, you can take a warm bath, but make sure the water isn't hot, or a warm shower, just be careful not to slip, as you are quite off balance at this point. If you back is aching, use a heating pad to help provide some relief, but do ensure that you cover it with a towel, to keep from getting too hot. Do not take an aspirin or ibuprofen, as these increase the risk of hemorrhaging during labor, and only take acetaminophen if you have received the okay from your practitioner. Remember, however, not to lie on your back!

If you feel hungry, eat a light snack, but nothing that is heavy or hard to digest, as this can compete with the progression of labor. You may also want to avoid acidic foods, such as juice that may upset your stomach and induce vomiting later on.

You should also keep track and time your contractions from the beginning of one to the beginning of the next for about a half an hour, if they seem to be less than ten minutes apart. Don't make yourself crazy over the situation or become a constant clock watcher, as this can increase stress and anxiety levels. Sit back, relax and wait for the next phase of labor, as it is on its way.

Phase Two – Active Labor

Typically, active labor is shorter in duration compared to early labor and takes an average of two to three hours, although this number can vary drastically from woman to woman. As for contractions in active labor, they will be coming on more and more often, reaching about three to four minutes apart, will be stronger and get more accomplished in a shorter period of time.

Contractions will typically last anywhere from 45-60 seconds during active labor and you will notice a distinct peak in the middle. During this time, your cervix generally dilates to about 7 centimeters and you have less time to relax in between contractions, and will most likely be at the hospital or on your way.

As contractions progress during active labor, you may find it very uncomfortable to move around, experience increased pain in your back and legs, feel exhausted, have an increased bloody show and possibly be unable to talk during contractions, depending on the level of pain you are experiencing. Now is the time, also that your water may break, if it hasn't already, or your practitioner will break it for you.

Emotions may be at an all-time high at this point. Your mental state can range from excited that it's almost over, to feeling as though the pain is never going to end. You may be considering use of pain medications at this point and would need to talk to your practitioner about what's right for you. There are various methods of pain medication, which are discussed in the Q&A section, that can be used to provide relief during labor and delivery.

If you attended birthing classes, now would be a good time to start practicing the breathing techniques you learned. As each contraction comes on, you will need to begin breathing appropriately. This will help keep your blood pressure from raising too high and keep you from passing out, due to holding your breath.

You may be feeling thirsty, and with the permission of your practitioner, you can drink clear fluids to replace those you lose during labor. You may also eat a light snack, again with the permission of your practitioner, if you are feeling hungry.

Even though contractions are coming on pretty strong, you need to try and relax as much as possible in between them. This helps conserve your energy, which you will need for pushing in phase three – delivery. To relieve discomfort without pain medications, you may walk around, if you are able and make sure you urinate, even if you don't feel as though you have to. There is an increasing amount of pressure on your bladder and you may not realize you have to go, even though you do.

During active labor, you are likely to be at the birthing center or hospital, as was mentioned earlier. Not only will your spouse be there to coach you along, but you will have more nurses at your side than you can count. They will be there to monitor your progress, monitor your health and your baby's health.

It is likely that they will check your blood pressure routinely and monitor your baby through an electronic fetal monitor. They may also aide in timing your contractions, so they can put your practitioner on alert when you are ready for delivery. In the event you are not dilating, even with such strong contractions, they may need to help you along by using Pitocin. They are also your source for pain relief medications if needed. You will, by the end of this phase, move into advanced active labor, also known as transitional labor that prepares you for delivery.

Phase Three – Transitional Labor

You have now reached the most demanding phase of labor – advanced active labor, also known as transitional labor. The intensity of your contractions will increase dramatically, become stronger and occur about two to three minutes apart, lasting anywhere from 60-90 seconds. You will notice a peak in the intensity of the contraction, but unlike active labor, this will typically last the duration of the contraction. Dilation of the last three centimeters, to reach ten, will take place in a short period of time, anywhere from 15 minutes to an hour, on average.

At this stage, you may feel as though the contractions never completely dissipate and that you cannot relax in between them. You should, however, try and relax as much as possible, even though it may seem improbable. It is important that you hang in there, making it to the end, which doesn't take very long and soon you will begin to push, bringing your baby into this world.

It is a good idea to focus on how far you have gotten, as opposed to how much longer it's going to take. It is also important that you don't push at this point, unless you have been instructed to do so. Pushing before your cervix is completely dilated can cause it to swell and actually prolong delivery. To avoid pushing, because you will feel like you need to, try panting or blowing out air.

During this time, it is really important to practice the proper breathing techniques you learned in birthing class. Feel free to ask your spouse for help, as he is likely to be calmer that you, or ask the nurses for guidance. They have likely been in a labor/delivery room before and can guide you on your way.

Your nurses and hospital staff will continue trying to help you find comfort and provide support along the way. They will also continue to monitor your progress and monitor the condition of your baby and keep track of intensity and timing of contractions. If you have not already been moved to a delivery room, they will do this at this time, as sometimes labor rooms are separate than delivery rooms. Once you reach 10 centimeters, it will be time to delivery your beautiful, healthy baby boy or girl, making the last nine months, and possibly the last few hours of intense pain and discomfort all worthwhile.

Stage Two – Delivery of the Baby

Although it seems like you've been doing a lot during labor, up until now, most of the work has been conducted by your baby, your uterus and your cervix. Unfortunately, you have just been the punching bag they take out all the stress on. During stage two of labor and delivery, you will begin to work hard, pushing with each contraction at the guidance of a nurse or your practitioner, in an effort to delivery your baby.

You will be required to push in order to guide your baby through the birth canal and out of your body. Typically, this is accomplished in about 30-60 minutes, although some women have experienced very short delivery periods and very long delivery periods.

During this time, you will find that contractions are now coming at regular intervals, are about 60-90 seconds long, but do give you more time in between, somewhere around two to five minutes. It is also possible that the contractions are less intense and less painful. However, in some instances, they are slightly more painful.

There are a lot of different things happening with your body during this phase and your physical and emotional state can seem as though they are all over the place. You may go from having a renewed energy (second wind) to feeling complete exhaustion in no time. It is possible that you will notice an intense amount of pressure near your rectum, feel tingling sensations, burning sensations or stinging sensations around your vagina, particularly when the head crowns, meaning begins to show.

Emotionally, you may be feeling relieved that you can now begin to push or embarrassed, as a lot of people – nurses, doctors – will be standing around with their eyes on you in the direction of your vagina. It is important that you understand that delivering a baby is a common event for these hospital employees, and you need not to feel embarrassed – that have seen it all.

Depending on how long the pushing stage continues, you may feel slightly overwhelmed or frustrated that your baby isn't coming out as quickly as you would like him/her to. Do not feel as those you are an unfit mother, if at some point you aren't concerned with seeing your baby, but more focused on getting this event over with. This is a natural feeling, as your body has been through a lot during the last few hours, you are stressed, weak and exhausted. This will pass and has no reflection on the motherly love you will provide your baby with in the near future.

You will be required to get into a birthing/pushing position. This will depend on your practitioner and any specific hospital regulations regarding delivery. For the most part, women are on their back, with their legs lifted and separated. In many cases, a nurse, or your partner, will help you hold your legs back as you push with each contraction. This helps to open you up more, allowing the baby to come out easier.

With each push, it is important that you push with everything inside you, putting as much energy into each push as the last, if not more. This will help your baby move through the birth canal quicker. It is important to remember that you need to push with the lower half of your body and not the upper half. Think of pushing your baby through the birth canal in the same manner as you would move a bowel movement through your colon. It is very important that you breath and do not hold your breath while pushing. This can cause bloodshot eyes and black and blue cheeks from too much pressure in your face.

There is a chance, and you may have heard this, that you can force out anything that is in your rectum while pushing. This is a perfectly normal and common occurrence, and nothing that you embarrass you or inhibit the manner in which you push. You may also accidentally urinate while delivering, but that's okay. It is completely understandable and common, as there is so much pressure on your bladder and bowels at the time of delivery.

In general, you should do what feels natural, meaning push when you feel the urge, unless you are instructed not to. Take a few deep breaths, as the contraction becomes more intense, and when it peaks, take another breath and hold it, then let the air out slowly as you push with all your might. During each contraction, you may feel the need to push more than once, and this is fine, as long as your nurses or practitioner don't tell you not to.

If at any time you lose your concentration or urge to push, even though you should be pushing, your nurses and physicians will help coach you along. This is also a good time for your spouse to provide encouragement, provided you haven't kicked him out of the room by now.

It is also important that you follow all instructions of your delivery team. This includes not pushing when they tell you not to, in order to prevent the baby from being born too rapidly. You need to try and rest in between contractions when you are not pushing, so that you have energy for the next go-around.

In some delivery rooms, there may be a mirror where you can see the baby's head crown. It is important that you do not become frustrated if the head comes out and then disappears again. Delivering a baby is sometimes a two-steps-forward and one-step-back event. However, seeing your little one's tiny head, may just provide you with that renewed sense of accomplishment and energy you will need to continue pushing at the sign of the next contraction.

As the baby's head crowns, you will notice that some nurses come in and start preparing for delivery. They will be placing sterile drapes and arranging instruments, putting on surgical face covers and gloves, and sterilizing your vaginal area with antiseptic. In the event an episiotomy is necessary, which is an incision from your vagina area towards your rectum to help increase the size of the opening for your baby to come through, nurses will perform this procedure before the head crowns completely. Typically, this is conducted during the peak of a contraction, which increases the numbness in your vaginal area and is most often painless.

If your baby is not coming out easily on his/her own, your nurses may try vacuum extraction or forceps to help. Typically an anesthetic will be administered, if you do not have an epidural or other block already in place.

Once your baby's head is completely out, the nurses will suction excess mucus out of and away from the mouth and nose. They will then provide assistance in making sure both shoulders and the baby's mid-section, then feet are successfully expelled from the birth canal. Then, the nurses and practitioner will clamp and cut the umbilical cord (or have your spouse do this), and often they will lay your baby across your chest for you to hold for a few moments.

He/she will then be whisked away to be evaluated and rated using the Apgar scale at one minute and five minutes following birth. They will dry your baby off and take fingerprints and footprints for hospital records and attach a hospital bracelet to the wrist and ankle. They will then place an ointment in the eyes that prevents infections, weigh your baby, measure the length and wrap him/her in a blanket to prevent heat loss. They will then give you back your baby to cuddle, hold and admire.

Stage Three – Delivery of the Placenta

During the time the nurses are cleaning up your baby and getting him/her ready to begin bonding with you and your spouse, you will be delivering the placenta. You will continue to have mild contractions that last about one minute, as the uterus is separating the placenta from the uterine wall. Following delivery of the placenta, you may need to have some stitching if an episiotomy was necessary, but again, you likely won't feel anything.

In order to deliver the placenta, you will be required to push, even though you are likely exhausted. The nurses and practitioner will assist with this event and take care of any necessary stitching. Each hospital and/or birthing center has different policies on how this is conducted. Some may help by pulling gently on the umbilical cord while pressing and massaging the uterus to get the placenta to move out. Others may put pressure on the top of the uterus and tell you when to push, which also forces the placenta out. In some cases, Pitocin is used to speed up the process through an IV drip. This also helps shrink the uterus back to size and minimizes bleeding.

It is normal to experience bleeding, similar to that of menstruation following delivery. Your medical team will likely provide your lower half with a sponge bath to clean up an excess blood and fluid in an attempt to make you more comfortable. You will then be moved to your post-partum room and your baby to the nursery to have a complete pediatric exam conducted and a few protective procedures, such as his/her first round of shots.

While your baby is in the nursery, now is the time to get some rest. So that when he/she is finished in the nursery, you can relax and spend time bonding with your child, and starting the process of breastfeeding, if that is what you and your partner have chosen! Congratulations! You have just brought a new life into this world and deserve time to relax and enjoy your new baby!

Chapter 9 – What To Avoid When Pregnant

During pregnancy there are a few things you need to avoid to have a safe, healthy pregnancy for both you and your baby. From alcoholic beverages and tobacco use to illegal substances and caffeine, all pose a problem for you and your baby during pregnancy. Each category will be discussed in detail in this chapter, with the hopes that you will take heed of the advice and eliminate these unhealthy substances during pregnancy – if not for you, then for your baby!

Alcohol Consumption

For many women, drinking alcoholic beverages happens on occasion and sometimes you may drink a few too many here and there. While there is nothing wrong with that idea – for the most – you need to avoid alcoholic beverages while pregnant, as it can create a long, long list of complications for your unborn child.

With that said, there are women who have had a few too many while pregnant, although they did not know they were pregnant until several weeks later. Many women begin feeling guilty that they had drank after finding out they were pregnant. Fortunately, this is one concern that can be put aside. According to research, there really is no evidence that a few drinks on one, or more, occasions early in pregnancy can cause harm to a developing embryo.

However, this does not mean that if you suspect you are pregnant it is okay to continue drinking. The minute, or second, you discover or suspect you may be pregnant, you should avoid all alcoholic beverages completely. Understanding the effects of alcohol on an unborn child may help you put that bottle down – if you haven't already – a lot faster.

Alcohol enters the bloodstream of the baby in the same concentrations it enters the mother's bloodstream. Essentially, each alcoholic drink consumed is shared with your baby – not a good idea. Further, it actually takes the baby twice as long to remove the alcohol from the system than it does for the mother to expel the alcohol from her system. This means, that at about the time the mother is getting tipsy, the baby is to the point of passing out.

Heavy drinking is described as five or six drinks per day of any alcoholic beverage – wine, beer or distilled spirits. Unfortunately, this type of behavior during pregnancy can result in a whole host of complications for the baby and for the pregnancy in general. One of the most serious negative side effects of drinking alcohol while pregnant is the development of Fetal Alcohol Syndrome (FAS) for your baby.

This condition has been described as 'the hangover that lasts a lifetime' and presents many complications throughout life for the baby as he/she grows. Often, children born with FAS are undersized, mentally deficient and often present with deformities of many parts of the body, such as the head, face, arms and legs, heart and central nervous system. Further, drinking during pregnancy can result in death to the child.

Infants who survive FAS later show signs of developmental, learning, behavioral and social problems and often cannot make sound judgments. The sooner an individual quits drinking alcohol while pregnant, the less risk there is for the baby. On the other hand, the more you drink alcohol during pregnancy, the more at risk your child becomes for developing FAS-related issues and the risk of death.

Although heavy drinking is what leads to FAS, this does not mean that it is safe to consume even one or two drinks per day throughout pregnancy. This type of behavior has its own set of issues, such as increased risk for miscarriage, premature labor and delivery, complications during labor and delivery, low birthweight, stillbirth, abnormal growth and development and problems later in childhood.

You may hear rumors that one glass of wine per day is acceptable. However, this is not true at all. There may be an individual or two that have successfully drank a glass of wine per day and still delivered a healthy baby, but this does not mean that this is a safe assumption. In general, when it comes to alcohol drinking and pregnancy here's what you should go by – you do not need to feel guilty about what you drank prior to knowing you were pregnant, but as soon as you suspect pregnancy, eliminate all alcohol consumption from that point on!

While this may be as easily done as said for some, others may have issues with alcoholism, wherein they rely on alcohol to unwind and relax in the evening. For women who rely on alcohol, it is important that they focus their attention elsewhere and find other means for relaxation, such as music, a warm bath, exercise, a massage or reading.

There are also other alternatives, such as non-alcoholic beer, virgin – meaning no alcohol – versions of many drinks, such as daiquiris and sparkling cider to replace a glass of champagne at a wedding or other special event. Remember, your baby is the most important thing you need to focus on and taking care of yourself takes care of him/her.

Tobacco Use

Many women who are smokers or have been smokers in the past have questions regarding smoking during pregnancy. This section will explain the risks of tobacco use – particularly smoking – while pregnant, plus whether or not smoking in your past is harmful to your current pregnancy.

First of all, if you have used tobacco products, such as smoking cigarettes, in the past, whether you just quit a month before you were pregnant or ten years before you got pregnant, there is no need to feel guilty. There is no evidence that suggests your prior smoking habits will negatively impact your current pregnancy or unborn child.

With that said, however, it is very well researched and documented that smoking during pregnancy is very harmful to your baby. This is especially true if you continue smoking beyond the third month of pregnancy. It is, in fact, hazardous to your baby's health.

Smoking while pregnant causes your baby to be confined in a smoke-filled womb with no oxygen to breath. A baby's heartbeat will increase, they will begin coughing and sputtering and they will not be able to grow and thrive as they should be.

Further, smoking increases the risk for complications during pregnancy for the mother and the baby. This can include vaginal bleeding, abnormal placental implantation, ectopic pregnancy, premature placental detachment, premature rupture of the membranes and premature delivery of the baby. In fact, studies have shown that more than 14% of preterm deliveries are related to cigarette smoking of the mother.

If your baby is born prematurely, it is likely that he/she will be small, from having a low birthweight to being shorter in length. A baby that is born too small can be at risk for developing illnesses as an infant and puts them at risk for perinatal death, meaning death that occurs just before birth, during birth or right after birth. Smoking also increases the risk for your child to develop apnea, which means that they stop breathing and can be at an increased risk for dying from SIDS – Sudden Infant Death Syndrome.

Smoking during pregnancy can also result in deformities, such as cleft lip and cleft palate, not to mention small head circumference. As your baby grows, providing it makes it past infancy, he/she will be at an increased risk for complications throughout life. This can include long-term physical and intellectual deficits, respiratory diseases, ear infections, TB, food allergies, asthma, short stature, Attention Deficit Hyperactivity Disorder and an aggressive attitude. These issues are even more prominent when adults continue to smoke around the child as it is growing up.

This goes for letting individuals smoke around you when you are pregnant and letting people smoke around your baby or child as it continues to grow after birth. Second-hand smoke is just as bad, if not worse – according to research, as first-hand smoke. You should try and avoid being around an individual while they are smoking. The effects from someone else smoking can be just as bad as if you were smoking. Also, if it is your partner that smokes, please ask them to take it outside, so that you are not being surrounded by the smoke – remember if you are surrounded by smoke, so is your baby.

Lastly, just because someone you know successfully smoked and had healthy babies doesn't mean this is going to be true for you, nor does it make it acceptable for you to try it. Smoking puts a negative impact on your growing child. Taking a risk that could negatively impact your child just because another person was successful is not a good idea. It's kind of like this – you wouldn't go jumping off a bridge because that person didn't it and survived, because a life raft happened to be going by, so don't smoke just because it was okay for that person. Make your own judgments and choose the option of protecting your baby.

Sadly, there have been more than 115,000 miscarriages and more than 5,600 infant deaths that are all related to smoking while pregnant. Therefore, if you smoke and have discovered you are pregnant, it is recommended that you quit now. If you need help with quitting, talk to your practitioner. He/she will be able to provide you with tips and tricks to get you through. Some suggestions may include increasing fruit and fruit juice, milk and greens intake, and cutting back on meats, fish and cheeses. Eliminate caffeine, as it can add to the jitters, get more rest, and exercise, as it can provide a similar 'kick' that you used to get from smoking.

Drug Use – From Marijuana To Cocaine & Everything In Between

As you have learned, everything that you consume, inject, smoke, whatever the case may be – goes from your bloodstream to your baby's blood stream. This means that each time you take a puff of marijuana, snort a line of cocaine or give yourself an IV injection of meth, per se, you are sending these drugs directly to your baby, not to mention a mile-long list of complications.

Similar to tobacco use and alcohol drinking, there are absolutely no positive outcomes when using drugs while pregnant. There are, however, negative issues that result from using drugs, such as marijuana and cocaine while pregnant. For instance, marijuana use by the mother while pregnant can increase the risk of birth defects, damaged genes and cancer, as well as medical issues similar to those caused by Fetal Alcohol Syndrome.

With that said, there is no evidence that using illegal substances – or medical marijuana – in the past, prior to becoming pregnant, can have a negative impact on your pregnancy now. This does mean, however, that you should avoid using illegal substances or any other type of drugs while you are pregnant.

Further, it is important that you are honest with your practitioner about past drug use and current drug use, so that he/she is able to provide help for you and increase protection for your child. There is evidence that suggests even using drugs one time during pregnancy, particularly in the later months, can cause preterm labor and or death of the fetus.

Use of any drug while pregnant, unless prescribed by a physician who knows you are pregnant, is putting your child at risk for medical complications during pregnancy, during birth and afterwards. If you need help with your drug habits, discuss your situation with your practitioner to ensure a safe, healthy pregnancy.

Caffeine Use

Although not as harmful as alcohol drinking, tobacco use or use of illegal substances while pregnant, caffeine is still not a good idea. Caffeine, like any other substance that enters your body while pregnant, goes straight to your fetus and can have a negative impact on your pregnancy and your unborn child, such as miscarriage.

Research is still ongoing when it comes to the complete effects of caffeine use during pregnancy. There currently does not seem to be a risk associated with women who drink one to three cups of coffee – or other caffeinated beverage – per day. This is not the case, however, with an individual who drinks much more caffeine.

Either way, you do need to be cautious about the amount of caffeine you are consuming, as there are some other negative risk factors that could result in complications. For instance, caffeine is a diuretic-type beverage, meaning it draws fluid and calcium out of your body. Both of these are vital components of a healthy pregnancy and should be increased not decreased during pregnancy.

In addition, these beverages, especially when filled with sugar and cream, are filling and satisfying, but provide little nutritional benefit, if any. This means that you are filling yourself up to the point of not being hungry, when you really are lacking in the vital nutrients needed for both you and your baby.

There is also evidence to suggest that caffeine can increase mood swings, and prevent you from sleeping, even if it does not create these effects when you are not pregnant. This means that you will not get the adequate amount of sleep required during pregnancy, especially if you are consuming caffeine later in the afternoon.

Lastly, caffeine can interfere with the absorption of iron in your body. As you learned earlier, iron is an important part of pregnancy and if the caffeine you are drinking prevents iron from being absorbed, you could be at risk for complications associated with iron-deficiency. This can include developing anemia, increased fatigue and other issues.

If you cannot quit drinking caffeine completely, try reducing consumption to at least half of what you are currently taking in, unless of course, half would keep you above two-three cups per day! For the safety of you and your baby, it is recommended that you try and substitute healthy beverages that are decaffeinated for those you would normally drink with caffeine. Talk to your practitioner about adequate substitutes for caffeinated beverages.

Sugar Substitutes

Although many individuals believe that sugar substitutes help with weight control, they would be unpleasantly surprised to find out this is not the case. This is mostly because they are added to a variety of already unhealthy foods. You should use sugar substitutes with caution, especially during pregnancy.

There are a variety of different types of sugar substitutes that you should be aware of. This will enable you to know whether or not you should eat a certain product. Aspartame is probably the most commonly used sugar substitute and is found in most diet beverages. The others include saccharin, sucralose (Splenda), acesulfame-K, sorbitol, mannitol and lactose (milk sugar).

Before diving into foods containing sugar substitutes, it is important that you talk with your practitioner. He/she will be able to provide you with more advice on which sugar substitutes are appropriate for you during your pregnancy and which you should avoid.

Hot Tubs, Saunas & Electric Blankets

Although you don't necessarily need to take a cold shower while you are pregnant, it's also not a good idea to soak in a hot tub, bath or take a hot shower. You should also avoid using electric blankets while pregnant. This is because these items can increase your body temperature and anything over 102°F for too long is hazardous to the development of your unborn child. You should know, however that it takes about 10 minutes for your body to reach this temperature in water that is over 102°F, and can be quicker if the head and shoulders are in the water as well.

Having your body reach these high temperatures – and staying there for a prolonged period of time – can cause negative effects on you, thus harming your baby. When it comes to electric blankets and heating pads, specifically, although there is no evidence to support pregnancy difficulties related to their use, the theory is there and you should use extreme caution.

It is recommended that you find other methods for warming up if you are cold or heating an injury. You can use more blankets or cuddle up with your spouse to keep warm. You can use a warm towel or a microwavable bean bag heating pad that does not continue to stay hot for muscle relaxing. Further, it is never, never, ever a good idea to sleep with heating pads, as they can increase the risk of being burnt.

When it comes to harmful things to avoid, there really is a long list. If you are unsure if you should or should not use something or eat something specific while you are pregnant, it is always best to discuss the situation with your practitioner. He/she will be able to provide you with the most concise answers and how you should go about a particular situation and whether or not it is safe.

Chapter 10 – Q&A

There are a lot of subtopics when it comes to pregnancy and not all questions can be answered in one book. This chapter focuses on some important points and aspects related to pregnancy that were not necessarily included in the book, or maybe focuses on providing you with more details about a particular topic.

In the event your questions are not 100% answered here or in this book, it is best to talk with your practitioner. He/she will have all the answers you need to guide you along your way through a healthy pregnancy, labor and delivery. This book has just been a guideline, providing you with questions you can ask, and a basic understanding of pregnancy, labor and delivery.

When Is A C-Section Necessary?

You may have heard the term cesarean section, or more commonly, C-section, at some time during your life or maybe only during your pregnancy. There are typically certain circumstances that require a C-section delivery. It is important that you understand the reasons why you may need a C-section and how a C-section is conducted, and the differences between a C-section and a vaginal birth.

You should be aware that although history does not classify C-section deliveries as safe, they have proved to be as safe as vaginal deliveries, for both mother and baby. In some cases, where the baby is in distress or labor is not progressing, C-section are considered the best option as opposed to trying to continue with a vaginal delivery.

Unless this is your second pregnancy and you had a C-section the first time around, you will likely not know you will need a C-section until it happens. Typically, with the first pregnancy, a vaginal birth will be attempted and followed-through. However, there are times where a vaginal delivery can turn into a C-section and in some cases, what is known as an emergency C-section. This only occurs when the baby is in distress or the mother starts having complications that can progressively become worse with a continuing vaginal delivery.

With that said, there times when a C-section is scheduled. One reason is that you have previously had a C-section due to complications with a vaginal delivery attempt. This makes it possible for you to know when you will have your baby, be able to be a part of the delivery, and your spouse be a part of the delivery as well. In cases with emergency C-sections, this is not always possible.

A scheduled C-section may also take place if you have a medical condition, such as preeclampsia, that does not often result in a safe vaginal delivery for the mother or the baby. Talking with your practitioner regarding your concerns about C-sections is recommended. He/she will be able to provide you with information as how they will proceed if one is necessary and what you can expect.

What Does Rh Negative/Positive Mean?

During the very early stages of pregnancy, your blood will be tested to determine what type you are and whether or not you are Rh negative or positive. Being Rh negative can present some issues with your health and the health of your baby. Here's a little information on what being Rh negative means.

You inherit your blood cells from your parents and they are either Rh negative or Rh positive. Rh positive means they contain the Rh factor and Rh negative means the Rh factor is not present in the blood cells.

In the event you are Rh negative and your baby is Rh positive your body's immune system can view the baby as a foreigner and begin attacking the baby's immune system. This phenomenon is known as Rh incompatibility. However, it is impossible to determine what your baby's blood type will be until he/she is born.

With that said, one way to determine if it is possible for your baby to have Rh factor in their blood, meaning they could be Rh positive, is by the father's blood type. If your spouse's blood type is negative, then there are no worries, as the baby will have a negative blood type also, and will not be seen as a foreigner to the mother's immune system. If the baby's father is positive your baby could have positive blood, thus creating an incompatibility between you and your baby, when it comes to blood types.

Fortunately, if this is your first pregnancy it will not really negatively impact your child. However, in the event that some of your baby's blood enters your blood stream during delivery, this could pose a problem for consecutive pregnancies and your future children. You will need to prevent the Rh antibodies from developing, which is done through a series of two shots.

The first shot will be given at about 28 weeks during your first pregnancy, wherein you will receive a vaccine-type injection of Rh-immune globulin, which is known as RhoGAM. You will then receive another dose of RhoGAM within 72 hours after delivery of your first child, if their blood type is positive. In the event their blood type is negative, there is no need for a second shot.

Now that you know you are a negative blood type, you need to make sure that you get the RhoGAM shot with every pregnancy and be sure to have your baby's blood tested at birth, to determine if you need another. Most likely, your practitioner will be aware of the situation and take care of this for you, but it's always nice to have a heads up on situations such as this.

Is Making Love While Pregnant Safe?

Making love, or simply sex, is what got you pregnant in the first place, but you may be concerned about whether or not it is safe to continue having sex or making love now that you are pregnant. Many couples experience changes to their sexual interactions during the nine months that you are pregnant, particularly changes in sexual appetite.

For some women they become more willing and wanting to make loves, while others may find it uncomfortable or feel inadequate about the way their body is changing and looking and not find themselves attractive, thus eliminating a sexual drive.

In general, sex during pregnancy is different for every couple. You may find that it is better than it's ever been, which could be a result of heightened sensations in your vaginal area and the sensitivity of your nipples, or you may find that it is something you would like to enjoy but just can't.

If you and your spouse are a couple that continue to have a sexual appetite, you may be wondering if continuing with love making is safe for your unborn child. The answer is yes, as long as you are having a normal, healthy pregnancy and are not at an increased risk for complications, you can continue making love.

You need to understand that your fetus is well protected and cushioned inside the amniotic sac inside your uterus, which is safely secured and sealed off by the mucous plug that develops in the opening of the cervix.

Following intercourse, you may feel contractions that begin as a result of your orgasm. In a normal pregnancy, it is safe to assume that this will not initiate a miscarriage and you are not in danger of going into labor at any point. In fact, you may find it interesting that studies have shown that couples who continue to be sexually active during pregnancy have lower rates of premature labor, and an increased emotional connection to one another which creates a positive effect on the overall pregnancy.

All in all, having sex during pregnancy may be different from anything you've experienced in your lifetime. It is, however, perfectly safe and can be good for you, both physically and emotionally. It can bring you and your spouse even closer together, it can help you prepare physically for labor and delivery, as it strengthens your pelvic muscles and it is relaxing, which is good for everyone involved, even baby, who by the way, cannot feel (aside from the comforting rocking) or see anything you are doing. If you are still unsure whether or not making love is safe for you, discuss your concerns with your practitioner.

What Medications Are Used For Pain Relief During Labor?

One of the biggest concerns for any pregnant women, particularly if this is their first time being pregnant, is the use of medications during labor and delivery. It is likely that you have heard horror stories related to medications used during labor and delivery for pain relief.

However, you should talk to your practitioner about their use and safety, but you can learn a little about them here, where the facts are presented and not an opinion of what you should do, as that is totally between you, your spouse and your practitioner to decide.

Epidural Block

The most commonly heard of type of anesthetic used during childbirth is the epidural block. This is a regional nerve block that is used in both vaginal and cesarean deliveries, with more than 50% of women who give birth in hospital asking for one by name. The recent surge in deliveries with epidurals may be due to the relatively safe nature of the anesthetic, how easily it is administered and the patient-friendly relief it provides. An epidural block keeps you from feeling anything below the waist, including diminishing the pain felt with contractions. It can make you more comfortable, but has no effect on your mental status, and allows you to be awake during the entire delivery process.

Prior to an epidural being administered, your medical team will start an IV to prevent you from having low blood pressure. You may also have a catheter inserted in your urethrea, as an epidural can prevent you from feeling the urge to urinate, which is vitally important.

In order to administer an epidural, an antiseptic will be applied to your back, which will then be numbed using a local anesthetic. A larger needle will them be placed into the numbed area into the epidural space of your spine. Typically, while this is taking place you are required to lean over a table to steady yourself, or hold onto a pillow while in the sitting position and lean over, while a nurse helps hold you still. You may feel a slight bit of pressure or a tingling sensation while the epidural is put into place. The needle is then removed, while a catheter stays in place, providing you with a continual dose of numbing medication, which typically begins to alleviate pain within three to five minutes.

Most women find that they can still effectively push while the epidural is in place, but if pushing become a problem, as you cannot feel how hard or soft you are pushing, the epidural can be stopped to bring back a little feeling, giving you full control of the pushing process.

Regional Nerve Blocks

Next on the list are other types of regional nerve blocks. This includes a pudendal block, a spinal block or a saddle block. A pudendal block can be used to provide pain relief early in the second stage of delivery, but is most often not used until just before vaginal deliver occurs. It is administered through a needle inserted in the vaginal area and reduces pain in the vaginal area, but not in the uterus, meaning you will still feel contractions.

A spinal block is used for C-section delivers, allowing you to feel nothing from the neck down, but you are still awake. Sometimes this type of block can cause some nausea and vomiting. Typically, however, an anesthesiologist will remain in the room during a C-section to continually monitor your progress and provide extra pain relief and medications to reduce nausea and vomiting. A saddle block is typically used right before delivery when a vacuum extraction or forceps-assisted vaginal delivery is necessary.

Analgesics

More commonly known as Demerol, this pain reliever is the most commonly used form in obstetrics for labor and delivery. it is typically administered through a slow-dripping IV so that it can be monitored and quickly stopped if necessary. Demerol is typically not administered until labor is in full effect and there are no indicators that this is false labor.

When using Demerol, you may feel slightly fuzzy mentally, which some women do not like the feeling of. Others find it relaxes them and helps them cope with contractions better. Depending on your sensitivity to medications, you may experience nausea, vomiting, depression and a drop in blood pressure, all of which will be closely monitored by your nursing team.

What Causes Premature Labor & Can You Prevent It?

When you become pregnant, one of the scariest and saddest things to consider is that you will do something wrong that causes you to go into labor early, possibly harming your baby. You should know, however, that it is more common in the United States for babies to be born later than their due date, as opposed to before their due date, and those that are born early are typically

Although your chances of carrying your baby to term are high, you could still benefit from working to prevent an early labor. This can be done by following the advice and instructions of your practitioner, avoiding the things you should avoid during pregnancy, including tobacco use, alcohol use and drug use and provide your baby with adequate nutrition.

You can also help decrease your risk for preterm labor by not standing for long hours, and avoiding heavy physical labor. You have an excuse to sit down and watch people around you work – for once take advantage of this opportunity. Lastly, it is important that you make sure you are in good overall health. Have regular checkups with your dentist and contact your practitioner when you suspect any type of infection or illness is brewing, including a cold.

If you are very concerned with having preterm labor, discuss your feelings with your practitioner, he/she may be able to give you advice on what you can do to decrease the odds of this occurring and provide you with some additional tips on being healthy while pregnant. They will be aware of your medical history and health conditions, so they will be able to provide you with individualized options.

Is Exercising While Pregnant Important?

[This answer is for women who are at low-risk for complications and are having a normal, healthy pregnancy. If you are not one of these women, you should talk to your practitioner about whether or not exercise is appropriate for you and what types of physical activity you can participate in.]

Women who do not exercise during pregnancy often become less fit as the months go by, which is typically attributed to the excess weight you are gaining. Exercising can keep you in shape while you are pregnant and also help you from gaining too much weight while pregnant, especially when combined with the pregnancy diet.

Because exercise releases endorphins in your body, you are likely to feel more energized, both physically and mentally, sleep better at night, strengthen your muscle and increase your endurance. You will also benefit later in pregnancy from continuous exercise through your pregnancy, wherein as your belly begins to grow and becomes quite large by the ninth month, you will have better control of your balance and stability, which will decrease your risk for falling.

Further, exercising can reduce backaches, constipation, bloating and swelling. You will also find that if you exercise during pregnancy you will likely return to your normal size much quickly during post-partum recovery. Although you should talk to your physician about what types of exercise are right for you, consider participating in some type of the following activities – aerobics, calisthenics, light weight training, water workouts, yoga, relaxation techniques and pelvic toning. You should also make sure you are properly stretching before and after exercising and taking in adequate amounts of fluid.

What Is The Effect Of Cell Phone Use During Pregnancy?

Cell phones are a part of 99.9% of Americans' lives. However, there has been a debate about whether or not cell phone use during pregnancy is safe or not. Cell phones of the past have been known to put off harmful amounts of radiation, but typically do not cause harmful effects, unless you spend several hours a day on one.

Although the debate is ongoing, there is no clear evidence to suggest that cell phone use during pregnancy is safe or is not safe. However, risks with cell phone use seem to be limited to the user. There has been no link to birth defects or miscarriage simply from using your cell phone.

With that said, cell phones do pose one major risk to all, and those who are pregnant – driving and texting or talking is never a good idea. This task, although dangerous for anyone and illegal in some places, can be particularly hazardous to a women who is pregnant.

As you know, your pregnancy has somewhat left you absentminded, caused you to daydream, and decreased your focus on regular tasks. Try combining talking on the phone and/or texting while driving and you've doubled your chances for having an accident. If you don't already practice safe/smart cell phone use and driving, you should start now and keep it that way. If you need to make a call or send a text, pull over first, take care of business and then continue driving.

What Is Preeclampsia?

A common term heard during pregnancy is preeclampsia. The question is, however, what is it, are there any signs and symptoms and can it be treated. All of these questions will be answered for you, starting with the realization that preeclampsia is pregnancy-induced hypertension, or high blood pressure. You should also know that preeclampsia is often referred to as toxemia and can lead to eclampsia, an extremely dangerous medical condition.

This can be diagnosed by paying attention to the signs and symptoms, particularly swelling, high blood pressure and protein in your urine. As you know, these three things are checked at every office visit during pregnancy. Although your practitioner may not explain why he/she is checking these things, you can guarantee they are screening for preeclampsia in an attempt to provide you with a safe and healthy pregnancy.

Preeclampsia is diagnosed if after the 20th week of pregnancy your blood pressure is 140/90, or higher, especially in a women who has never had high blood pressure readings in the past. You may notice some swelling, particularly in the face and hands, with an sudden increase in unexplained weight gain, which is likely due to water retention.

If untreated, preeclampsia can lead to more complications, including very high blood pressure, blurred vision, fever, headaches, rapid heartbeat, confusion, pain in the upper abdomen, restlessness, twitching and abnormal kidney function, to name a few. When it comes to your baby, you need to be concerned about growth restriction and inadequate amounts of amniotic fluid. Fortunately, if you are visiting with your practitioner on a regular basis, as you should be, this will be caught early and treatment can begin. There are a multitude of treatment methods used for preeclampsia, but the only cure is giving birth, which you need to wait nine months for.

Because preeclampsia is essentially high blood pressure, treatment methods will be centered around lowering your blood pressure. This can begin with diet, exercise and stress reduction methods, but may result in the use of medication. If medication is used, it will likely be IV magnesium sulfate.

Many times, however, a person with preeclampsia is required to stay in the hospital until delivery day and be continually monitored. If you are allowed to go home, it is likely that you will have a nurse dropping by on a regular basis to monitor you in between physician visits.

In the meantime, it is important that you pay attention to signs and symptoms of your condition becoming worse. Pay attention to severe headaches, visual disturbances, rapid heartbeat and unusual pain in your abdomen. If these events occur, it is very important that you seek prompt medical attention.

Discuss concerns about preeclampsia with your practitioner to ensure a safe, healthy pregnancy for your baby. Further, you should know that if you did not have high blood pressure prior to pregnancy that you will return to normal following delivery. You would need to, however, be aware of signs and symptoms in later pregnancies, as you are now at an increased risk for developing preeclampsia again.

What Should You Know About Miscarriage?

Miscarriage is a scary word, especially for anyone who is pregnant, and is the reason why many women keep their pregnancy to themselves and their spouses until the first trimester is over. Early miscarriage happens for a variety of reasons, but can also be prevented, in some cases. Here's what you need to know about miscarriages.

If you have had trouble with an IUD in the past and have scarring of the endometrium you may have more difficulty getting pregnant. However, once implantation is well established in the uterus, miscarriage is not a concern. This is the same with abortions. If you have had an abortion in the past, you likely have scarring on your uterine wall. However, this will only affect implantation and not be cause for a miscarriage early in pregnancy.

You should also know that a heated argument, or temporary increase in stress does not cause miscarriages. Although a minor accident or injury cannot cause a miscarriage, serious injury can, which is what makes wearing seatbelts in the car and being extra cautious more important.

Further, myths that physical activity, carrying your older children, hauling in groceries, lifting moderately heavy objects, and participating in sexual intercourse (unless your physician advises against it) does not cause miscarriage.

With that said, there are events and habits that can increase the risk of having a miscarriage. This includes poor nutrition, smoking, insufficient hormones, hormonal imbalances, infection, such as bacterial vaginosis, some STDs and chronic medical conditions, such as severe kidney disease, congenital heart disease, diabetes and thyroid disease.

However, once these risk factors are identified, they can be monitored and controlled to decrease your risk for having a miscarriage. It is important that you discuss your complete medical history – leaving nothing out and being completely honest with your practitioner – so that these conditions can be controlled.

In addition, there are some medical conditions that lead to miscarriage and cannot be changed, such as a malformed uterus, uterine fibroids, and other chronic illnesses. If you have concerns about miscarriage, it is best to discuss them with your practitioner. He/she can give you advice and guide you in an effort to prevent miscarriage when possible.

Are Household Cleaning Products Safe To Use During Pregnancy?

Many women are concerned about the effects of different household products on the baby during pregnancy, particularly those used in cleaning. With that said, many household cleaning products have been used for decades with no proven link to causing harmful birth defects or complications during pregnancy. This means that it is highly unlikely that you would be compromising the health of your baby by scrubbing a toilet or polishing your furniture. In fact, the elimination of the bacteria in your home by using cleaning products can actually reduce the risk of infection to both you and your baby.

There has been no evidence or tests that suggest that the temporary inhalation of household cleaners while tidying up pose any threat to your baby. You should, however, clean with care and be careful of the products you are using. Make sure that you avoid potentially hazardous chemicals. Here are a few tips on things to avoid, but you can also get a list of harmful chemicals from your practitioner.

If a cleaning product has a strong odor or fumes, make sure you do not breathe them in directly and make sure you are cleaning in an area with adequate ventilation. If this is not possible, do not use this product and leave that cleaning to your spouse. Pump-type sprays are always preferred over aerosol-type spray and are better for the environment.

One thing you should never, ever do, even when you are not pregnant, is mix ammonia with chlorine-based products. This creates a toxic fume develops in the form of chloramine gas and is deadly, to say the least. Other toxic chemicals that you should avoid are those used for oven cleaning and dry-cleaning, as they clearly have warnings that they contain toxic chemicals.

If you do find the time and the energy to clean while pregnant, make sure you wear rubber gloves. They help prevent the absorption of harmful, toxic chemicals through your skin. Anything that is absorbed in your skin goes through your bloodstream directly to your baby.

Aside from household cleaning products, there are a few other things you should steer clear from in your environment. Lead is a big one, and as you may have heard, heavy exposure to lead can reduce the IQ levels of children, but also poses negative risks to a pregnant mother and her unborn child. Problems from lead exposure can range from minor birth defects to serious behavioral and neurological problems as your child grows.

Insecticides are another toxic chemical you should avoid during pregnancy. While it is good to grow your own garden, having fresh fruits and vegetables while you are pregnant, using insecticides in your garden, in your home or around your home could pose a threat to your unborn child, such as birth defects.

Whenever possible, try to take a natural approach to pest control. In the garden, try using a forceful stream of water from the garden hose or use a biodegradable insecticidal soap, which is safer to use. Inside the home, use traps that draw bugs in and trap them, as opposed to spraying all sorts of chemicals throughout your house, that could cause side effects.

You should also know that even insecticide products that are labeled 'natural' are not necessarily safe either. In fact, they often contain boric acid, which is harmful when ingested or inhaled and is particularly irritating to the eyes.

Although you really want to get decorating and designing your child's room, leave the painting to your spouse. Even though paints produced today do not contain lead and there is no evidence to suggest that it could cause your baby harm, you never know what may turn up in the future regarding paint fumes. There is no need, when someone else can do the painting, for you to be subjecting yourself and your baby to possibly harmful fumes.

What Is Gestational Diabetes?

As was described earlier, you will be required to take a glucose-screening test somewhere around the 28th week of pregnancy, which is standard procedure during pregnancy. It was also explained that this test is used to discover whether or not you have developed gestational diabetes as a result of your body changing from pregnancy.

Gestational diabetes is a temporary form of diabetes in which your body quits producing adequate amounts of insulin needed to remove excess sugar – glucose – from your body. If detected during these tests, monitored and controlled, gestational diabetes poses no risk for yourself or your growing baby.

However, in the event that you do not monitor your blood sugar, the excess sugar circulates through your blood and into the fetal bloodstream, causing complications and risk for both mother and baby. Uncontrolled gestational diabetes can put you at risk for having a large baby and developing preeclampsia, which is pregnancy-induced hypertension.

There are cases in which gestational diabetes is found earlier in pregnancy through your monthly urinalyses conducted at every visit. You may also notice that you are increasingly thirsty and an increase in urination, accompanied by fatigue. As you know, increased urination and fatigue are normal pregnancy symptoms, which is why it may be difficult for you to realize that this is due to gestational diabetes.

Treatment of gestational diabetes involved extreme control of blood sugar levels, which are easily accomplished through medical and self-care. You will need to have your blood sugar levels tested routinely during pregnancy to ensure that your gestational diabetes is under control. You will need to follow a diabetic diet, make sure you do not gain excessive amounts of weight during pregnancy, exercise according to your physician's orders, get plenty of rest and make sure that you are taking any medications prescribed by your practitioner how they prescribed them.

If you have any questions regarding medications prescribed or how you should be taking them, it is important that you speak with your practitioner, to ensure you are not doing anything that could be potentially harmful to you or your baby. You can prevent the development of gestational diabetes by eating a balanced diet, making sure you are at a healthy weight prior to pregnancy and practice good exercise habits. Furthermore, studies have shown that obese women can reduce their risk of gestational diabetes by 50% simply by adding an exercise routine to their day.

What Are The Benefits Of Breastfeeding?

There is an ongoing debate about whether or not children should be breast fed or formula fed. Here are some benefits to breastfeeding your baby and how it can also benefit you.

Benefits To Baby

There are several reasons why breast milk is the best food source for your newborn. First of all, it is made solely to satisfy the nutritional needs of your baby. There are near 100 ingredients found in breast milk that are absent from cow's milk. As much as commercial baby formulas try to duplicate these ingredients, they so far have not been able to. Formula is made from caseinogen, a major protein found in cow's milk. In contrast, lactalbumin – the major protein found in human breast milk, is more easily digested and more nutritious than its bovine counterpart. Although the fat content in the two milks is quite similar, human milk fat breaks down more easily when digested and used by an infant. This easy digestion allows important nutrients to be more easily absorbed by the baby as well.

Constipation is rarely an issue with breastfed babies. This is because breast milk digests more easily. Diarrhea is also less common in breastfed babies than in formula-fed babies. There are certain diarrhea-causing organisms that are no match for breast milk. Also, breast milk encourages the growth of beneficial flora located in the digestive tract, which does many good things for the body including further reduction of stomach upset.

Allergies and infections are a tough match for breast milk. There are few babies that are actually allergic to breast milk, although they may have an allergic reaction to something in their mother's diet – including cow's milk. In contrast, it is this cow's milk with its main protein found in baby formula, which can cause mild to severe allergic responses. Often times, formula-fed babies are immediately switched to soy formula when they cannot handle regular cow's milk formula. This soy formula is even further in composition from breast milk than cow's milk is, and can also cause its own type of allergic reaction.

One of the main arguments for breastfeeding is that it lowers the risk of infection in a baby. This includes ear infections – something otherwise common in children. There are a variety of other diseases that have been shown to have a lower risk in breastfed children as well, thanks to the transfer of colostrum and other immunity boosters from mother to baby.
Studies have shown that breast feeding tends to equate to a lower risk of being overweight as an infant as well as a lower risk of obesity later in life. Although studies aren't finite, there is also research pointing to lower cholesterol levels in adulthood.

A baby's mouth might benefit from breastfeeding as well. The baby needs to put more effort into sucking from a breast than from a bottle, making stronger jaws, teeth, and palate. There is also a lower risk of cavities later in life for those children that were breastfed as babies.

It has been found that breastfeeding might also raise a child's IQ. This is because of DHA (brain boosting fatty acids) found in breast milk, as well as the intimate relationship between mother and baby that fosters the intellect of a developing young brain.

Benefits To You

Unlike store-bought baby formula, human breast milk is safe, assuming the mother has been avoiding drugs and alcohol. This gives many nursing mothers peace of mind that they are feeding their baby something trustworthy. Baby formula can be contaminated, prepared improperly, tampered with, or have an expired shelf-life. It is also completely free of cost.

Many moms, depending upon whether they are pumping or strictly feeding from the breast, tout the convenience of breastfeeding their babies. The breast is always available as long as the mom is available, and it is at the right temperature. However, for moms who work outside of the home, pumping and storing is required, which means just as much work as for formula feeding mothers.

Breastfeeding mothers also appreciate the fact that postpartum recovery occurs more quickly than if they were not breastfeeding. When babies suck on the breasts, a hormone called oxytocin is released. It is this hormone that speeds the shrinking of the uterus back to the size it was pre-pregnancy. Some women even experience quicker weight loss since breastfeeding consumes calories, although they should be supplementing for the calorie loss in their diets.

There are not many women who look forward to their periods returning after childbirth, and breastfeeding can also delay this inconvenience. It can take up to four months for a breastfeeding mother to start menstruating again, as opposed to two months for a formula feeding mother.

Besides the conveniences of breastfeeding, there are also health benefits to the mother. One of which is strengthening of the bones. Nursing encourages mineralization in the bones, which can benefit a woman even after menopause. Women who tend to take in enough calcium and are generally healthy may reduce the risk of bone fractures if they breastfed their children earlier in life.

Weight Gain During Pregnancy – What You Need To Know

It is a no-brainer for pregnant women that they should expect to gain weight during their pregnancy. But questions naturally arise. How much weight is normal? Will I lose it all? At what rate should I be gaining weight? Can I eat whatever I want? How quickly can I lose the weight after the baby is born?

How Much Should I Gain?

Every woman is different and so are their bodies and metabolisms. Stressing too much about weight gain during pregnancy is not healthy, but it is also not healthy to be too relaxed either. Too much and too little weight gain can both have a negative effect on the baby and on you. The amount of weight you should gain while pregnant is somewhat dependent on how much you weighed pre-pregnancy. This is a topic to discuss with your practitioner. Keep in mind, the weight gain is not just that of a 7 lb. baby. There is amniotic fluid, breast tissue, blood volume, placenta, water weight, and maternal storage of fat to be considered as well.

Typically, the formula for how much weight to gain revolves around your body mass index, or BMI. This magic number is calculated by multiplying the number 703 by your weight in pounds and then dividing the product of that calculation by your height in inches squared. A woman with a BMI between 18.5 and 26 is usually advised to gain anywhere between 25 to 35 pounds. This is considered average. Anyone with a below average BMI is usually advised to gain more weight than the average 25 to 35 pounds, and anyone with an above average BMI is usually advised to gain less. Mothers carrying multiples are advised to gain even more. It is important though to consult your practitioner despite anything you may read or what your peers might tell you.

Risks associated with too much weight gain include difficulty in assessing the growth of the baby if there is too much fat in the way. Added pounds also equate to discomfort and risk of injury. Preterm labor, gestational diabetes, and hypertension are risks to both the mother and baby during pregnancy.

If a woman gains too little weight during pregnancy she may deliver prematurely, have a baby with low birth weight, and suffer from restriction of growth in the uterus, amongst other problems. These babies tend to be more prone to sickness as well since their bodies have not had the chance to grow and develop as they should.

Unfortunately, even having this weight gain goal in mind does not mean your pregnant body is on board with your goal. Morning sickness and food aversions or cravings tend to interfere with the well-intended goals of a pregnant woman. A pregnant woman's activity levels need to be considered as well. A sedentary office worker with no other children at home who does not exercise will need to consume fewer calories than the mother of four who is on her feet all day.

At What Rate Should I Be Gaining Weight?

Slow and steady wins the race. This is best for both you and your growing baby. The rate at which a woman gains weight while pregnant is just as important as the pounds gained themselves. A sporadic delivery of nutrients and calories to the baby is not as healthy as a consistent and sufficient supply would be. A gradual weight gain also helps the mother by allowing her body to make slow adjustments to weight gain and the physical strains that accompany pregnancy. One example is stretch marks, which are less likely to occur if the skin does not have to make sudden stretches. Pounds tend to be shed more quickly postpartum when weight gain is gradual as well.

A steady weight gain does not mean that the weight should come gradually over 40 weeks. The baby grows at different rates throughout the pregnancy, and is so small during the first trimester that it really needs minimal weight gain during that period.

During the second trimester, the baby grows much more quickly and your appetite should increase. During this time frame, months four through six, you should expect to gain one pound to one and a half pounds per week. Keep in mind that this only an average recommendation.

The third trimester sees the baby gaining weight rapidly, but this does not mean that your weight has to increase as rapidly. If you were gaining one and a half pounds per week during the second trimester, expect to gain one pound per week during the third, while your baby keeps growing. Some women see a tapering off of their weight gain during the last month or even lose a few pounds since their stomachs do not have as much room to accommodate large meals.

A general rule of thumb is to monitor your weight throughout your pregnancy to make sure you are near the above mentioned targets. Any concerns about too rapid weight gain should be discussed with your practitioner since dieting during pregnancy is never recommended. Gaining more than 3 lbs. in one week during the second trimester or more than 2 lbs. in any week during the third trimester is a reason to check with your practitioner, especially if you have not been overeating nor had sudden changes to your diet that would trigger such rapid weight gain. You should also consult your practitioner during months four through eight if you see no weight gain for more than two consecutive weeks.

How Do You Know If You're Having Twins?

During recent years, there has been a 50% increase in the number of twin births in the United States. Even more amazing is that the number of multiple births (triplets or more) has increased by 400%. This may be due to the fact that women are having babies at older ages, meaning that they are using fertility treatments that tend to bring an increase of multiple births. Also, women over the age of 35 are more likely to release more than one egg during ovulation because of increased fluctuation of hormones. Another surprising discovery is that researchers are finding that women with BMI's higher than 30 pre-pregnancy are more likely to have fraternal twins than women who have BMI's under 30.

If you are one of the women who have been blessed with a multiple birth, you most likely have fears and concerns. You may even wonder if your body is capable of carrying more than one child. Rest assured that you are more than capable and so is your body.

How Will I Know?

The first proof of evidence of twins is in the ultrasound. Different circumstances my prompt your practitioner to do an ultrasound early in your pregnancy but for the most part, the most accurate way to detect twins is after week 12. Any sooner than that and one baby may be hidden. However, even sooner than with the ultrasound, a Doppler can detect two heartbeats if the practitioner knows what to listen for as early as the 9th week. It is at that point that an ultrasound may be ordered in order to verify the findings.

It should be no surprise that more babies equate to a larger uterus. At your prenatal visits, your practitioner will measure your fundal height to measure your baby's (or babies') growth. If it seems larger than normal, this may be another indicator of twins.

Sometimes women who are carrying twins experience more pregnancy symptoms than women carrying one child. This is sometimes due to an increase in the pregnancy hormone, hCG. However, this is not to say that anyone experiencing extreme nausea should assume they are carrying multiples.

Fraternal or Identical?

Once you find out that you are having twins, you will most likely be curious as to what kind of twins you are having – fraternal or identical. Fraternal twins result when two eggs are fertilized simultaneously. There are two placentas, one for each baby, with fraternal twins. These are the most common. Identical twins are less common and result when one fertilized egg divides and splits into two separate embryos. They may have their own placentas as with fraternal twins, or they may share one.

Choosing a Practitioner

If you are pleased with your normal ob-gyn, there may be no need to consider finding a new one just because you are carrying twins. However, you may feel more at ease knowing that he or she has dealt with multiple births before and knows how to treat them. For example, twins tend to be delivered before the 40 week mark, since it is sometimes safer for the mother and her ever expanding body to deliver between 37 weeks (considered full-term) and 40 weeks. You will want to discuss their policies on induction and how far they will allow your pregnancy to progress to make sure you are on board with their decisions.

You will also be spending more time with your practitioner if you are carrying twins, since they require a little extra care. If you aren't completely happy with your practitioner, it may be wise to find one that you feel more comfortable with since they will be seeing a lot of you during the 9 month time frame.

Weight Gain

The recommended amount of weight to gain when carrying twins is different than that of a single pregnancy. Mothers of multiples should plan on consuming an extra 150 to 300 calories daily, per fetus. This does not mean consuming empty calories (sugar and carbs) however. Protein, veggies, fruits, beans, and some dairy are of course recommended over an extra serving of ice cream or French fries. Make your calories count and they will benefit both you and the baby, as well as make it easier for you to lose all that weight after the babies are born.

Water and iron are also not to be ignored when carrying multiples. Even mothers with single births sometimes experience low iron levels. There is a dramatic increase in red blood cells when pregnant and they need iron in order to do their job. A lack of iron results in anemia, which can be adjusted with an iron supplement should your practitioner find that your iron levels are low. Mothers of twins are also at an increased risk of dehydration, so drinking water is very important – at least 64 ounces daily.

Delivery

Your twins may pose quite the commotion during delivery depending on their positions in the uterus and the timing of labor. Approximately half of all twin births are vaginal. The remainders require a C-section (cesarean). The reasons may vary but usually have to do with the mother's and the babies' health. Sometimes C-sections are planned and sometimes they are not. It is important to know what to expect to some extent when going into labor with twins, but also just as important to be able to "go with the flow." This is why it helps to have a practitioner with whom you have a trusting relationship and who knows the importance of your birth plan so they can stick as close to it as possible without jeopardizing the health of you and your babies.

Deliveries tend to take longer with twins, which may come as no surprise. Sometimes the practitioner has to reach into the birth canal to remove the second baby who was not quite as ready to come out as the first one. For this reason, many mothers of twin births choose epidurals, but this is a personal choice. Do not assume that just because you are having twins, you have to have an epidural.

Recovery

For the most part, the recovery process for mothers with twins is the same as for those with single births, however, the rate at which recovery occurs is slower. This is due to the fact that their bodies have been stretched farther than they would have with a single birth, and they may have been much less active during the last few months due to the discomfort of carrying multiple babies. And extra weight equates to extra aches unfortunately, even after delivery. Still, the process of recovery is no different than with a single birth. The major factory in recovery will be whether you had a vaginal birth or a C-Section, which requires more time to heal.

The most important things to remember when carrying twins are to maintain a regular relationship with a practitioner that you trust, take care of yourself, and expect the unexpected. No matter how much you want your birth to go a certain way, it is more important to consider the health of you and your babies. This means being flexible and able to listen to the advice of your practitioner in the delivery room.